IN CARE
A STUDY OF SOCIAL WORK
DECISION MAKING

JENI VERNON & DAVID FRUIN

NATIONAL CHILDREN'S BUREAU

In Care
A Study of Social Work Decision Making

© *Crown copyright 1986*

SBN 902817 25 6

Published by
National Children's Bureau
8 Wakley Street
London EC1V 7QE.
Telephone: 01-278 9441

Typeset in Great Britain by
Getset (BTS) Ltd
6 Mill Street
Eynsham, Oxford

Printed by
David Green Printers Ltd
Newman Street
Kettering, Northants

Contents

Contents

Acknowledgements

This study was one of a series commissioned by the Department of Health and Social Security and formed part of the department's rolling programme of research with the National Children's Bureau.

Our thanks are due to the DHSS for funding the study, to the Research Liaison Officer, Jenny Griffin for her unfailing support and encouragement and to members of the department for their helpful comments on an earlier draft. Our thanks, too, to Tilda Goldberg and Chris Payne who likewise commented on an early draft. Many colleagues and ex-colleagues at the Bureau have contributed to the project: for his help in the preparatory stage, we should like to acknowledge the part played by Peter Wedge, formerly Deputy Director at the Bureau, and for her assistance in carrying out the fieldwork, we are grateful to Janet Sayers. Frances Laidlaw has typed almost all the material relating to the project and we thank her for the patience and equanimity with which she has typed successive drafts. We are also indebted to Ron Davie, Ken Fogelman, Roger Fuller, Lydia Lambert and Peter Riches for their helpful comments at various stages. We extend a particular 'thank you' to Janet Lewis whose arrival at the Bureau coincided with the start of writing up the project: her contribution has been immeasurable.

Finally we extend our gratitude to the staff of the eleven anonymous social services departments who participated in the research, and particularly to the social workers who gave so generously of their valuable time. We apologise in advance if at times we appear unduly critical of their work: our concern to promote the interests of the children in their care does not mean that we have failed to recognise that most workers are highly committed and caring individuals carrying out their unenviable task as best they can.

Jeni Vernon
David Fruin

CHAPTER ONE
The Research in Context

In 1977 the Department of Health and Social Security commissioned the National Children's Bureau to undertake research examining factors affecting the length of time children spend in care. Key questions identified by the Department were 'What circumstances determine how long children stay in care?', 'How is the decision to (or not to) discharge a child from care taken?' and 'How long does a child need to be in care to be regarded as permanently in care?'.

The initiative for the research arose in response to mounting concern during the earlier part of the decade about the quality of public care of children separated from their families. For example during that period a number of research reports were published each suggesting the need for a critical reappraisal of selected aspects of the child care service. Research by Packman (1968) and by Davies, Barton and McMillan (1972) showed that there were large, seemingly unaccountable, variations between local authorities in terms of the provision of child care services and the numbers of children in care. Likewise, deficiencies in the two principal types of accommodation for children in care continued to be reported. For example, whilst the number of children in residential care continued to rise, Prosser (1970) in her research review of residential care concluded that 'in terms of bringing up children in circumstances that approximate most closely to those of a normal family, residential care would seem to offer the most costly and least beneficial alternative' (page 25). The writer in her second review of fostering studies (1978) felt that the conclusions of her first review published 12 years earlier still held: 'That the number of placements which breakdown is too high, and is damaging to children' (page 39).

Widespread public concern about the care system was stimulated by the succession of child abuse cases, beginning with the death of Maria Colwell, and tug of love cases involving contests between natural and foster parents over the custody of children in care. The detailed reports of the inquiries following such cases, particularly those concerned with child abuse, highlighted the difficult decisions involved in child care and whilst 'the overall impression of practice given by the reports is one of much good work', they also revealed 'numerous omissions, mistakes and misjudgements by different workers at different times' (DHSS 1982).

Increasingly, then, the capability of local authorities to 'parent' the children in their care was called into question and doubt was cast on whether there were any positive aspects of admission to care. In particular, the findings of Rowe and Lambert's 'Children who Wait' study (1973) contributed to this notion. According to Morris (1984) this report 'rocked the social work world and particularly those who had been relatively complacent about the quality of child care services offered at that time in Britain as a whole'. The study drew attention to the large number of children who appeared to be drifting in local authority care without firm plans being made for them. On a national basis, some 7,000 children were estimated to be in need of a foster or an adoptive home. The researchers further showed that once children had been in public care more than six months, they had only a one in four chance of leaving before they were 18, that only one in ten children had any contact with their natural parents after six years in care, and 41 per cent had no contact with a parent at all.

Despite the depressing picture presented by the Rowe and Lambert study and the many local authority studies which followed it (for example Bainbridge, 1973; McGrath, 1977), we in Britain had very little information about the length of time children spent in care, far less why. Somewhat surprisingly, prior to 1976 the system for collecting national statistics on children in care did not include information on duration in care. Nonetheless the available statistics did show that whilst the number of children *in* care was generally rising throughout the 60s and early 70s, the proportion of children entering care was decreasing. A trend of more children remaining longer in care was indicated, but it was not apparent why.

It is to this latter question — why children remain in care — that this study addressed itself. However, before proceeding to detail the approach we adopted, it is only appropriate to point out some of the developments in the provision of the child care service which began to occur at approximately the same time as the research and continued throughout and beyond its duration.

At a central level, the DHSS attempted to take an active role in improving practice: guides to adoption (1970) and to foster care practice (1976) were published. A number of circulars were issued providing local authorities with guidelines for procedures and practice in the field of child abuse and research was commissioned not only on length of time in care but, for example, into variations in local authorities' willingness to admit children to care and the consequences, and the difficulty of maintaining links between children in care and their families.

On the legislative front the Houghton Committee report on adoption (1972) led eventually to the Children Act 1975. This Act not only promoted the local authority adoption service and instituted changes in the existing adoption legislation but included directions to local authorities (and courts) on their conduct vis a vis children in care. Sometimes referred to as 'the Children's Charter', the Act was not wholeheartedly welcomed in all social work quarters, some commentators feeling that the philosophy of the Act would lead to the infringement of parents' rights (see for example, Holman, 1976). By placing on local authorities the duty 'to give first consideration to the need to safeguard and promote the welfare of the child in care throughout its childhood', what the Act did clearly imply was the need for sound and careful planning in dealing with children.

This theme was also pursued in the professional literature of the period. As a result of the findings not only of the 'Children who Wait' study but also of American literature (Maas and Engler, 1959; Bryce and Ehlert, 1971), the permanency principle emerged and was promoted. As Morris (1984) points out: 'Most writers (Brown 1974, Pringle 1980, Neilson 1976, Adcock 1980a) stress the importance of permanent homes for children as a developmental need, and in consequence as a right'. On the broad practice front, the most evident effect of the permanency principle has been the move away from residential to foster care, a movement which according to Curtis (1981) represents a diversion of the findings of 'Children who Wait'. According to her 'They (the findings) are not seen as showing to what extent we allow children to grow up without the permanent security of a family they can call their own. Instead, they are interpreted as showing the need for children in care to be fostered, rather than left in institutions. The implications are not understood in many social services departments'.

Although a number of commentators have identified the propensity to place children in fostering rather than adoptive situations (for example, Turner, 1980), there were considerable developments in the adoption field. Apart from the legislative changes of the 1975 Children Act which overall facilitated the adoption process, groups of children were identified as 'hard to place' and in consequence specialised adoption agencies were set up. The Parents for Children adoption agency in London, Barnardo's New Families project and the New Black Families

IAS/Lambeth Project, to name a few, represented attempts to provide permanent homes for the older child in care, the mentally or physically handicapped, family groups of children and children from ethnic minority groups.

During the course of the study, then, developments were underway which arose in response to the same concerns about social work practice as led to the commissioning of this research. In conducting the research we have been aware of these developments and anxious to note their influence on the wider child care front. Our observations on this and our resulting conclusions form the major part of this report. In a sense, however, concern about the care offered to children has, if anything, heightened in this country over the past few years and the policy and practice recommendations to central government of the Short Report (1984) highlight the increased expectations of practice today. Whilst the picture of practice presented by our report is undoubtedly depressing, it is to be hoped that it may, in some small way, contribute to developing improved ways of serving the interests of children in care.

Our approach to the research question

Prior to the mid-70s much of the research in this country had focused on identifying factors predictive of admission to care (see for example Schaffer and Schaffer, 1968; Mapstone, 1969; Holman, 1970; and Wedge and Prosser 1973), an approach which led to the conclusion that there were few, if any, measurable family and child characteristics which consistently and usefully predicted admission to care. None of this research addressed the question of length of time in care. In the United States, a number of research studies were carried out (see for example Jenkins 1967, Murphy 1968 and Fanshel 1971) specifically looking at a variety of demographic variables and their links with the length of time children spend in care. Although individually they identified what appeared to be significant factors, their rather inconsistent findings overall suggest that local community and/or agency factors may have a significant bearing on duration in care.

For this reason we agreed with our sponsors to discount an approach which relied heavily on quantitative data about children and their families and as such underplayed the contribution of the agency factor. From an early stage, then, our own approach was to examine the process of the child's career in care. This entailed considering the questions

'Why do some children return home?', 'Why are some adopted?', and

'Why do some remain in care?', not in terms of child and family characteristics, but in terms of the role of the agency responsible for children in care *vis-a-vis* different outcomes.

Obviously the range of agency characteristics which may interact with client characteristics in affecting what happens to a child is wide. Such characteristics include for example, the legislative framework within which the service offered by the agency is defined, as well as the skills and personality of the individuals employed by the agency to undertake day-to-day work with the client. Accepting the need to refine our approach from this global perspective, we were subsequently influenced by material from a number of disparate fields.

First, given the concerns about the quality of service to children in care and their families which gave rise to this piece of work, we considered studies of service delivery to client groups. Although there were no specific studies of service delivery to the child care group, the start of the research coincided with the publication of 'Who Cares'? (Page and Clark 1977), a Bureau development project. This report drew attention to the negative feelings of many young people about their own care experience and in particular highlighted the deficiencies in planning for children. As one young person put it elsewhere 'I thought they had all sorts of plans about what should happen to me, and I was bloody angry because they wouldn't tell me. When I got older, I realised that nobody actually had any plans at all. That hurt me and made me even more angry'. (Quoted in Parker, 1971 page 50).

In addition, writers dealing with other client groups (see for example Goldberg *et al* 1970 and Bayley, 1973) had indirectly commented on the quality of planning in social services. They expressed concern that social workers could deal with cases for not inconsiderable periods of time with no clear aim or objective in mind. Whilst many explanations have been offered for the resulting crisis-orientated approach, (for example, shortage of staff, lack of resources, high proportion of untrained staff), the implications of such studies, when transferred to the child care field, were that there was a likelihood that local authorities rarely had plans for the children in their care.

Our attention was therefore drawn to the planning and decision making function in child care. As we have already mentioned, the 1975 Children Act formally highlighted this function as a responsibility of each local authority. Likewise the professional literature of the period consistently drew attention to the need to make plans for children in care.

Parker, perhaps the most forceful exponent of the need for explicit   5 planning in child care, has argued over a number of years (notably in his 1971 lecture, Planning for Deprived Children) for a rational and explicit planning approach to clients, assisted by predictive techniques developed from the improved collection and analysis of information. Planning for children, he defines, as 'having a reasonably clear practical view of the future we wish for them, and more specifically, taking a sequence of steps which is instrumentally relevant to that end (page 13)'. Parker's general views are shared by most other recent commentators. The DHSS Working Party on Fostering Practice (1976), for example, states firmly: 'The responsibility of care agencies to make and carry out individual plans which meet the needs of children entrusted to their care cannot be over-emphasised' (page 139).

In similar vein, Adcock (1980b) urges that there should be 'a realistic discussion at an early stage about long-term future plans' (page 17), whilst Cooper (1980) writes: 'As soon as the child comes into care a period of assessment may be needed . . . a sound plan should then be made for the future' (page 27).

Such literature emphasises, then, the responsiblity to take decisions and make plans on behalf of children and indeed urges these activities as a priority for each local authority. Nonetheless there was little evidence at the start of this research that this was a documented policy of any one local authority.

In addition, research in the field of organisation studies has indicated that whilst in most organisations, decision making is organised so that the most significant decisions tend to be concentrated at higher levels, in welfare organisations one can argue that a substantial part of agency policy is not necessarily defined as such by some form of senior management group, but consists of 'an aggregate of individual decisions made by individual workers' (Hall, 1974). Smith (1965), describing such an agency, made use of the concept 'the frontline organisation', a primary characteristic of such an organisation being that the locus of organisational initiative is to be found in frontline units, a feature described by Smith (1970) as 'a dispersal of power'. Lipsky (1980) in describing the same types of organisations refers to them as 'street level bureaucracies', which he defines as public service agencies employing a significant number of people who interact directly with citizens in the course of their job. These employees he refers to as street level bureaucrats and they, like the frontline units in frontline organisations are considered to have 'substantial discretion in the execution of their work' (page 3). Lipsky further comments on the inherent tensions of those street level bureaucracies which attempt to retain accountability of frontline workers '. . . bureaucratic accountability is virtually impossible to achieve among lower level workers who exercise high degrees of discretion, at least where qualitative aspects of the work are concerned'.

On the basis of such literature, we concluded that a significant factor in determining the length of time children spend in care might well be the process by which decisions were made about their future. The aim of the study was therefore to examine the context in which such decisions are taken and plans are made and to consider the factors which influence these. Given, also, that the majority of such decisions appeared to take place at the interface of the agency and client, i.e. at the level of the social worker handling the case, we decided that this should be the focal point of our research.

The research design

Beyond this, the basic components of our research design were influenced by three factors. First we felt it fundamental that our eventual research style should enable us to understand the actions and behaviour of those involved in decision-making in child care. At the same time, however, we were aware that there was likely to be a wide range of practices and policies amongst individual workers, teams and departments and wished to avoid findings which were not generally applicable. On the one hand an intensive study in a limited number of areas was indicated and on the other a larger scale more impressionistic survey. Secondly, we viewed decision-making in child care as a process occurring over a period of time in which decisions and events are multiply determined by the past and in turn affect the future. To be understood, such a process needs to be followed over time, prospectively as well as retrospectively.

In considering these factors, we recognised that our material needed to be firmly anchored to a defined and potentially replicable sample of cases or events, that it needed to be collected longitudinally and from across a broad spectrum of authorities. Thus from an early date in the study we agreed to examine decision-making in child care by following, in a number of different areas, the care careers of selected children over a period of time. Third and finally, because of the overall complexity of our subject matter — decision-making — we felt that our understanding could only be enhanced by obtaining data from as wide a variety of sources as possible. We did not therefore rely exclusively on any of the conventional approaches but made combined use of case records, interview data from social workers and observations.

With these general ideas in mind we spent some time in a number of authorities experimenting with target sample numbers, construction of the sample and overall data collection techniques. As a result of this and a subsequent pre-test, we were able to determine the number of local authorities with whom we would work, the number and methods for selection of children who would form the basis of our sample and to finalise the data collection methods.

Selection of areas

In consultation with the DHSS we agreed to include eleven local authorities in the study to ensure coverage of DHSS planning areas, type of local authority, urban and rural areas and authorities with high and low proportions and numbers of children in care. In order to concentrate our resources, we agreed to cluster the samples of children by selecting them from one area office in each local authority. The local authorities were chosen by using DHSS local authority statistics on children in care and the classification of English personal social services authorities by Imber (1977). Our final list of authorities included three metropolitan districts, five counties, one outer and two inner London boroughs. Unfortunately, at the time, no standard information was available for each area office in England. However in the counties in which we worked we were able to specify particular area offices using Webber's and Craig's (1976) district level cluster analysis. In the metropolitan districts and London boroughs particular areas were chosen in consultation with senior officers of the social services department concerned. In general, we tried to work with a 'typical' area office for each department and at the same time attempted to obtain a balance of socio-economic areas across all sampled departments. In the event, 12 area offices participated since the rate of children entering care in one office was such that we had to include another to ensure our numbers in the allotted time.

Selection of children

In selecting samples of children to follow for a year, our intention was not to study the children themselves but that the children's cases would serve as entry points and tracers to identify related processes of decision-making. Our primary concern was with these processes, not with gathering information about groups of children or attempting to evaluate outcomes.

During the preliminary stages of designing the project, we experimented with numbers and construction of the sample. For example, we contemplated structuring the samples of children in a complex way according to their age, sex, legal status and placement as well as length of time in care. It became apparent, however, that such were the numbers of children in care in any one area office that we could not hope to achieve more than a few broad groupings of children. Thus only age and length of time in care were ultimately considered.

Furthermore, for the purpose of the study, we defined children in care as children either admitted voluntarily under the then Section 1 of the Children Act 1948 (irrespective of whether parental rights and duties had been assumed by the authority) or committed by the courts to the care of the local authority under one of the sections of the Children and Young Person Act 1969. Excluded from the study were children in care under other statutes, under Place of Safety Orders or being cared for by the local authority on an explicit 'holding' basis such as court-ordered remands, although some children, of course, had in the past or were to become in the course of the study, subject to one or more of these legal classifications.

In fact, two distinct sub-samples of children were used. One, known as the *into care* sample, was drawn from six local authorities and comprised children from the point of their admission to care, who were then followed for a period of at least one year. Eight children under 11 years of age and eight 11 years and older were planned to be drawn from each authority but in the event the combined total from the six authorities was 85.

The other sample, known as the *in care* sample, was drawn from five local authorities, including the pre-test area. In this sample all children in care under the above mentioned legislation on an agreed date were defined as comprising the area child care population. This population was divided into four sub-groups according to age (under 5 years, aged 5-10 years, aged 11-16 years and aged over 16 years), and then in each sub-group, the children were rank ordered by the time they had so far spent in care and, in order to ensure a spread of lengths of time in care, every n-th child was selected. Four areas each provided 21 cases in this manner and the pre-test 16, giving an overall total of 100 children who were again followed for a period of at least one year. An important modification to this basic sampling scheme was employed when a child was excluded if he or she would have constituted a third study child for a participating social worker.

Data collection — techniques and instruments

Our preliminary work had confirmed that neither our subject matter — decision-making processes — nor our main information suppliers — social workers lent themselves to a highly structured research style. Observation and 'informal' interviewing would have to play a significant role. Nonetheless since two researchers were to be actively involved in the fieldwork, some degree of standardisation was required and, anticipating later analysis and interpretation, it was felt advisable to structure as much as possible of the material as it was obtained. Furthermore there was a diversity of data to be collected from a wide variety of sources; whilst the data we ultimately sought were qualitative, as opposed to quantitative in nature, they depended on the receipt of factual information. Thus, whilst this was to be a prospective study, some basic knowledge of events in the past was desirable to aid our understanding of the present. As far as possible, then, we attempted to devise discrete sets of data collection instruments for the different types of data.

For the more factual information, four schedules were designed: a Child Information Schedule, a Case File Schedule, an Event Record and a Review Progress Record. The Child Information Schedule recorded basic information about the child, collected at the start of the research period from the case file and from the social worker, and was updated throughout the research period in the event of change. The Case File Schedule broadly comprised the background history of the case as obtained from the child's file. The form itself was only completed in the early stages of following a case and as a method of setting the scene for the first social work interview but its general format was also followed at subsequent stages of the research to prime the researcher about the topics to be covered in the next interview.

The remaining two instruments in this category were very much one page proforma. The Review Progress Record was begun at the start of the research and was updated throughout the period, basically monitoring dates by which reviews should be carried out, actual reviews occurring and whether these took the form of meetings or not. Finally, the Event Record was intended for recording basic information about significant events which the researcher would have to follow-up in interviews. Such events were difficult to pre-define beyond change of placement and legal status but in practice obviously covered a multitude of situations. Completion of the Event Record proforma was dependent on what was occurring on a specific case and for some cases, no such proforma was completed, whilst in others, a substantial research file built up.

Over and above the collection of material relating to sample cases and their associated sequences of events and decision making processes, the researchers gathered information about policies and practices affecting the handling of cases of children in care for each area office. With the exception of one authority, we were also able to arrange to receive copies of the social services committee papers for at least a twelve-month period to provide some useful background data about the authorities' policy making above the level of the local area office.

However, the main methods we were to employ were interview and observation and here it must be stressed that the schedules were primarily designed to serve as aids to the researchers in the topic areas to be covered and as a means of recording the information we were given. Basically there were to be four interviews with social workers on each child's case.

For the first interview, a lengthy schedule was devised which covered the social worker's perceptions of the child's admission to care — why and how this occurred, why the child was currently in care and the social worker's plans for the future, including the likely duration of care. Minor differences were necessary for the schedules used in the two sub-samples of children because of the different entry points to the child's care career, but this was largely a matter of emphasis.

We felt that at subsequent interviews with the social worker no single schedule was likely to satisfy the variety of situations which we might expect to have to cover and therefore no recording schedule was designed. Rather, our approach was to attempt to discover what had been happening on a case prior to a subsequent interview and to construct an individual 'one-off' interview schedule. In this sense, whilst our initial social work interview took the form of an 'in-depth interview', subsequent interviews are more appropriately described as focused interviews (Merton and Kendal, 1955).

The interview provided opportunities to focus on specific events (or non-events) but throughout the period the researchers also occupied what can best be described as an observational role. We did not for example, rely exclusively on the social worker's definition of an 'event' or a 'decision' but were alert to other influences and changes in a case

11

and to how these came about and were dealt with by the social worker. As far as was possible such observations were noted in the research file.

Our role in relation to formal meetings held on cases was more directly observational. Whenever possible, we attended these and a schedule was devised for recording the basic information about these meetings as well as our own less tangible observations on their outcomes. Where we were unable to attend, the form was partially completed from any documentation in the child's file, the interview with the social worker and from a knowledge of subsequent events.

Data were collected during the period 1978-81.

Data analysis

At the end of the fieldwork phase, we were in possession of a vast quantity of information recorded on a case-by-case basis which required synthesis in order for us to be able to generalise about decision-making in a broader sense.

To achieve this, we first embarked on a content analysis of the individual files. Two simultaneous exercises were involved. On the one hand, the information on individual cases was synthesised on to specifically devised sets of analysis forms organised according to topic: child information, planning information, formal and informal decision-making. At the same time, the researchers built up a list of emerging themes.

Negotiating access and research impact

Before concluding this introductory chapter, mention must also be made of the preparation which had to be taken in a study such as this, which placed high demands on the time of its subjects; and also of the likelihood of research influence where the same subjects were in repeated contact with researchers on specific cases.

In so far as obtaining the goodwill and collaboration of area staff was concerned, our approach was to ensure that each individual was provided with the opportunity of determining whether he/she wished to participate or not. In other words, whilst we generally met with senior management officials when first approaching a department, we emphasised that we sought only their agreement in principle to the research being undertaken in the department. We then attended area or team meetings to explain the research and outline the level of work required of those who might decide to take part, prior to asking for voluntary participants. The method appeared to be successful. Only one social worker refused outright to participate and many more than those who were ultimately involved, made themselves available for selection.

The issue of research impact is less readily resolved. With the small numbers of diverse cases and the absence of control groups we are unable to give a definite answer to the question: 'Did you affect the very process you sought to study?' What we are able to say, however, is that to the surprise of many of the social workers involved, they enjoyed the interviews; and being interviewed was not the threatening experience they had anticipated. A number further commented that they found the interviews to be of value in the sense that:

> It makes you think about the case . . . it makes you spell
> it out to yourself really why you are actually doing something.

> That was good . . . we don't often get the chance to sit down and talk
> to anyone about a case for this long.

Comments such as these evoked anxiety for the researchers lest they be influencing courses of action. Questioning of the social workers did not, however, suggest that this was the case and we concluded that, as is so in most interview situations, the respondent, the social worker, was deriving a sense of satisfaction from having participated in this process. One cannot, of course, discount the possibility that the line of questioning opened up new avenues of thought to the worker. The extent to which this constituted an impact on the case and the magnitude and direction of such impact on individual children s cases is difficult to assess.

We were aware of an impact in certain instances. This appeared to take the form of speeding up a plan which the social worker had already outlined. For example, in a very few cases, the social worker opened a second or subsequent interview by stating:

> You've had an effect here. I realised I hadn't done anything about this
> since last we spoke and so what I've just done is . . .

More commonly, no such direct reference was made but it was apparent that action had been taken just prior to the interview, suggesting that knowledge of the impending interview had served as a spur to action. On

13

the other hand, we did note that in many cases plans involving having to take some action were reiterated in successive interviews, suggesting no such impact on individual cases.

On the question of impact on the general process of child care, we are, if anything, more confident that our presence had very little impact. For example, review meetings were indefinitely postponed despite our involvement. In addition, there was an overt recognition on the part of the staff of the departments that since we were to be involved in the office for a period of not less than a year, any additional effort put on for our behalf was unlikely to be sustained.

To this extent, then, we ourselves are satisfied that our presence did not unduly alter the process we were following, and whilst it may have had some impact on individual workers in specific cases, this does not negate the validity of our overall findings. Furthermore, we felt encouraged in this viewpoint when later, at feedback sessions, staff at area level were able to identify with our general findings.

Summary

In a period of mounting concern about the quality of service provided by the child care system, the DHSS commissioned the National Children's Bureau to undertake research investigating factors affecting the length of time children spend in care. On the basis of research and professional literature both in this country and the United States, it appeared that the most fruitful line of enquiry into this topic lay not in examining the characteristics of children and their families but the context of decision-making in child care, who takes the important decisions and what influences them? For this purpose, a prospective study was carried out in eleven local authorities in England, to examine the decision-making process in respect of the care careers of 185 children of varying ages and length of time in care.

The format of the report.

In the next chapter the areas, the social workers and the children participating in the research are described, and subsequent chapters discuss the results. Chapter Three looks at the care careers of the 185 children in the study, with particular regard being given to length of time in care. Three admission types are identified with corresponding patterns of care duration. The next two chapters consider the decision-making aspect of admission to and discharge from care, who takes these decisions and on what basis. Chapter Six looks at the overall planning process in child care, whilst in Chapter Seven the role of different meetings and procedures in relation to planning and decision-making is explored. The penultimate chapter focuses on remaining in care and finally we summarise the findings and consider their implications for the child care service.

CHAPTER TWO
The Areas, Social Workers and Children

In designing the research, one of our concerns was to take steps to ensure that the context of the decision-making and planning which we ultimately studied could be viewed as a broad cross-section of the national picture. For this reason, we paid particular attention to the selection both of the authorities in which the research was to be conducted and of the children whose cases provided our basic data. This chapter, therefore, provides an outline of the areas, the social workers and the children involved in the study.

The local authorities

The eleven authorities finally participating in the study included three metropolitan districts, five counties and one outer and two inner London boroughs. They represented seven of the ten DHSS planning regions and in terms of Webber and Craig's (1976) general classification of local authority districts, the study areas covered all six 'families', with each area coming from a separate cluster. Imber's classification (1976) of social services authorities is more directly relevant to this research: the eleven sample authorities covered six of her eight major groups, including the extreme 'under' and 'over' spenders, and also spanned the range of scale of need for children's services.

Detailed comparisons for the combined eleven authorities with national totals were carried out. Overall the total number of children in care in the eleven authorities, as a proportion of their under 18 populations at 31st March 1979, was 6.81 per 1,000, a proportion not significantly different from the corresponding national figure of 7.73 per 1,000. Figures for the individual authorities varied from three cases of under five per 1000 to two with over 10 per 1000. Furthermore, in terms of legal status, sex ratio, age group, type of accommodation and duration of care episode, the figures both for children entering care and for children already in care in the 11 sample authorities differed little from the comparative national figures. In general terms, then, the eleven authorities can be considered as a representative sample of the 108 social services departments in England, forming in fact a close approximation to a representative 10 per cent sample of all English local authorities.

The area offices

As indicated in the previous chapter, there are no national figures summarising the salient characteristics of area offices and, in the absence of such standard information, it is difficult to establish with any certainty the representativeness of the 12 area offices participating in the study. From our own general experience of social services departments, we feel that none of the offices would be unfamiliar to social workers. Furthermore, from the information below it will be apparent that in terms of resources, structure and organisation the areas differed, suggesting we obtained a broad spectrum of 'type of office'. It should, however, be stressed that these distinguishing characteristics were not criteria on which areas were selected. Thus, while they may well have affected the nature and balance of the service provided in any one area, we have not attempted systematically to compare areas or to measure differences. However, where it appeared to us that area characteristics were significant to the handling of individual cases, we refer to this at the relevant stage of the report.

The catchment areas served by the offices were diverse in terms of their socio-economic features: a large and a small city each with a heavy industrial economic base; a small town manufacturing area; an over-spill estate; an area of rapid growth; a resort and retirement centre; a relatively well-off suburb; a regional service centre; a deprived, multi-ethnic inner city district; one of London's East End boroughs; and a new town. The sizes of the catchment areas ranged from one of approximately 10,000 to one of almost ten times that size, with the majority serving populations of between 40,000 and 50,000. Likewise, the size of the offices in terms of staff numbers varied from one with an establishment including administrative back up of less than 12 persons to another where staff numbers exceeded 40. The premises in which these staff were based included a wide range of buildings: a number were in converted, older houses, including a once-elegant small mansion; several were in purpose built accommodation; while others occupied somewhat drab space in shopping precincts and office blocks. Few were described as fully satisfying the accommodation needs of clients or staff, fieldwork staff often operating from noisy and very over-crowded conditions.

With the exception of one office, which was primarily organised on the basis of client grouping, all the offices were further sub-divided into geographical teams. At the outset of the study, six of the offices operated some form of duty rota system to process incoming work, whilst the remainder were divided into an intake and one or more long-term teams. In the course of the study period, and largely in response to fieldworkers' wishes, three of the areas operating duty systems changed to intake systems and two operating intake systems changed to patch systems.

Other than a commonly expressed criticism of the limited range of resources for adolescents, there were surprisingly few remarks about lack of resources for working with children and families. Nonetheless there did appear to be quite marked variation amongst the areas in the general availability of certain types of resource. For example, the authority of which one office was part was nationally recognised for its day care provision for children, another for its use of financial aid to families. Three areas operated family aide schemes, and in two the existence of NSPCC special units afforded the opportunity of professional collaboration in intensive work with families. In a further area a nearby advice centre was considered to absorb many of the general enquiries usually presented to the social services department and in another, a residential unit was available to undertake rehabilitative work with entire families.

All-purpose procedure manuals were available in most of the offices and, of particular relevance to this study, set out the official procedure governing the admission of children to care — the forms to be completed, the signatures required and the procedures for obtaining a placement. One of the twelve area offices functioned as a 'mini' department, offering all the services and functions of the department, with members of staff within the area being responsible for the management of residential and domiciliary services as well as those of fieldwork.

More commonly, the offices were fieldwork units, members of staff having to liaise with the authority's headquarters for the provision of many of the resources significant to work in the children's field. For example, with the exception of this one office, residential resources for children were centrally managed and administered. Officially, the procedure in obtaining a residential place was for the social worker to contact this central section. In practice, many variations to this procedure were found, involving the social worker making independent representation to specific establishments before or at the same time as an approach to the residential section.

The adoption service, too, was centrally located and, in general, operated separately from the fostering service. Adoption was viewed as a specialised type of work, adoption specialists not only providing adoptive placements but themselves being involved in the overall adoption work of the department. It was, indeed, rare for an adoption case to be dealt with exclusively at the area level, and more usually the case was transferred from the area to the adoption section.

The manner in which fostering resources were organised and managed differed widely from authority to authority and sometimes within authorities. At the start of the study, eight authorities operated centralised fostering units. One of these changed over to an area-based system in the study period, a further operated a dual system, and in another the area office with which we dealt was the only one in the authority to retain its local fostering officer after a department-wide change to a central service. In the remaining five authorities with central units, and in the three with area-based fostering officers, lists of foster placements and a description of them were supposed to be generally available. It was reported to us, however, that these were rarely maintained, and social workers had to rely on the knowledge of the fostering officer if there was one and failing that, on numerous telephone calls to check on availability.

In concluding this description of the offices, mention should also be made of the fact that the period of research fieldwork (1978-81) coincided with a time of cut-backs in public expenditure. Thus, amongst other things, actual staff numbers at area level were generally lower and sometimes considerably lower, than establishment quotas. Unfilled vacancies and frozen posts were features common to all offices and meant that on occasions most were under considerable strain in attempting to maintain operations and standards of service. In some, frequent, if short-term, reorganisations were initiated at the local level: area managers acted temporarily as team leaders and vice versa, the hours of being open to the public were restricted and new cases, including those of children admitted to care, were not allocated to social workers but 'held' by team leaders and district managers. In other areas no such local attempts were made to deal with the altered position.

It is likely this financial climate reinforced the area, as opposed to departmental, identity evident in each of the offices. Indeed, Satyamurti (1981) has already drawn attention to the importance of the area grouping in providing a reference group for area team members and in structuring standards of practice. Here we noted that references to 'the department' were often made in antagonistic terms, whilst use of the collective 'we' tended to be reserved for referring to the area office group. Area identities were, nonetheless, not always positive. A significant feature in constructing the positive or negative identity of the area appeared to be the extent to which the social workers in the area felt area management were 'in touch' with the circumstances of social workers' work. For example, although social workers in areas where steps had been taken in the light of the economic situation often expressed guilt about what they viewed as a reduction in the service to the client, the areas were nonetheless characterised by a relatively high level of staff morale. On the other hand, areas where the staff felt they were left 'to muddle through' were characterised by general discontent and unhappiness. The classic features of staff 'burn out' (Cherniss 1980), for example high levels of sick leave, staying in the office etc, were much in evidence in these areas in particular.

This then was the setting in which the processes of planning and decision-making which we studied occurred. We now describe the main actors in this setting, those holding the child care cases.

The social workers

Since our method of case selection was child-based, the involvement of individual social workers in the study was dependent on the selection of one of the children for whom they were responsible. In addition one of the criteria for selecting cases was that ideally no social worker should have more than two cases subject to research scrutiny. Our method of selection thus tended to under-represent social workers with large caseloads and conversely over-represent those with smaller case-loads.

In fact, it was not always possible strictly to adhere to the aforementioned selection criteria throughout the study period. In some instances, and where the social worker was willing, a third child on the caseload was included to allow us to complete a sample quota. Similarly cases were transferred during the study period, and this occasionally meant that for some time, some social workers were carrying more than two study cases. The most any individual social worker carried at one time was four cases. It should also be noted that not every social worker involved with a sample case was interviewed in the study year, cases being transferred between interview dates. This was not, however, a major problem: most of the *in care* cases remaining with the same social worker throughout the study period, and the majority of the *into care* cases being subject to no more than one change of worker.

Background data were collected on 114 separate social workers who were interviewed about the total 185 child care cases, this information being summarised in Table A2.1.

The majority (74 per cent)of those interviewed were designated main grade workers whilst 18 senior case workers or team leaders held responsibility for cases at least once during the study year. Rarely were social work assistants or students assigned responsibility for child care cases, a measure of the allocation priority given to children's cases since, on a national basis, social work assistants formed 15 per cent of field level social work staff.

The majority (72 per cent) held a professional qualification in social work and most had several years post-qualifying experience. Overall some two-thirds of the staff had three or more years experience, with two-fifths having more than five years experience. Only six of the 114 social workers were both unqualified and had less than a year's experience.

The general picture presented by these figures is of child care work being carried out by workers who combined experience with professional training. Furthermore, although the vast majority of these workers described themselves as generic social workers, not having a specialist caseload, it was apparent from their caseload figures that whether or not they were officially designated 'specialist', their caseloads were heavily weighted towards work with children and families. Of those designated 'social worker', caseload numbers varied from 20 to almost 50, with most having caseloads around 30. Cases involving work with children and families accounted for at least three-quarters of these caseloads, although, of course, the proportion concerned specifically with children in care could be considerably less. Whilst, then, it is appreciated that under the titles 'Child care work' or 'Work with families' is subsumed a wide variety of client situations and social work skills, the social workers involved in the study did not correspond with the popularised stereotype of the generic social worker struggling to cope with the demands placed on them by having to deal with the whole range of social services department clients.

The children

Since the overall numbers of children involved in the study was only 185, the numbers in particular groups were rather small for making detailed comparisons with national data. The limited comparisons made were based on DHSS data for children in care 1978-9 and one significant and substantive difference shown from the national data was in the under fives *in care* group. Here there were more children in care under Children and Young Person Act orders than would be expected either from the aggregate of the eleven authorities or the national picture. Examination of the sample in detail shows that the 'excess' of care orders principally arose from two non Metropolitan counties, and was in turn a feature which affected the distribution of episode duration: in the under fives in care group there is a relative under representation of children in care for less than six months and a relative over representation of children in care for between six months and a year. However, with the exception of this one sub-group, analysis indicates that overall both the *into* and *in* care samples may be considered substantially representative of their corresponding national populations at the time the study was carried out.

Given the wide range in ages and other features of the individual cases that we studied, there is no 'typical' case or even 'typical cases' that it would be worthwhile presenting. In subsequent chapters reporting the findings of the study, detailed case examples are used to illustrate specific points. Here we provide only some basic data collected at the start of the study on the children comprising each of the sub-groups in both sub-samples, indicating also the numbers in each sub-group who remained in care continuously throughout the study.

The 'into care' sample

The 22 children in this sample aged under 5 years, comprised equal numbers of boys and girls, six having been in care on at least one occasion in the past. Just less than a quarter were of non-white or mixed race origin and almost half were from single parent households or homes disrupted by divorce and separation. Half (10) entered care as part of a sibling group, only two on the order of the court and with one exception all were placed in foster care. At the time of admission, six of these children were described as being significantly behind in their development. Eight of the 22 remained in care throughout the study period.

The 18 children aged *5 to 11* years similarly comprised equal numbers of boys and girls but almost half (8) had already been in care, five on more than one previous occasion. A similar proportion to those *under 5* years came from 'disrupted' households, most were white and just under half were described by their social workers as 'disturbed'. Again half (9) entered care with siblings, two-thirds (12) on a voluntary basis under the Children Act 1948 and the same number (12) were placed in foster care. One-third (6) of these *5 to 11*-year-old children remained in care throughout the duration of the study.

The sub-group of 45 children aged *11-16* years at the time of their admission to care comprised twice as many boys as girls, almost a third (13) having been in care in the past. Approximately a quarter (12) were of non-white or mixed race origin and in seven instances some form of physical or mental handicap was reported. Behaviour difficulties typified this group, there being as few as five of the 45 cases where no reference was made to such a problem. Unlike their younger counterparts, more than half (25) of this sub-grouping were compulsorily admitted to care and only two in the company of siblings. Five of this older age group were fostered on admission, the remainder being placed in some form of residential care, primarily observation and assessment centres. More than half these children (27) remained in care during the whole of the study period, three remaining in their original placement, but seven having three or more placement changes in the year.

The 'in care' sample

Twenty nine children were aged *under* 5 years at the time of the their inclusion in the study, 18 boys and 11 girls. Of these, half (14) had been in care for less than a year, and a similar number (12) had been in care for two to four years. The majority came from white backgrounds but as with their counterparts in the into care sample, most came from disrupted families. One child was severely multi-handicapped and a fifth of the children (6) were described as being behind in their development. The majority (24) of children in this group had been admitted to care alone, often as very young babies. By the start of the study, 20 were subject to care orders, six of these having been made on the basis of evidence relating to other children in the family and, in six of the nine cases not subject to a court order, the local authority had assumed

23

parental rights and duties. Half (14) the group had contact with their parents or a parent on at least three or four occasions in the year prior to the study. Most (21) were in some form of foster care, four were placed home on trial and few (4) had experienced any placement change. Twenty-two of these 29 children remained in care throughout the study period.

The 26 children aged between 5 *and 11* years at the start of the study period comprised slightly more boys than girls. Most had already been in care some time: three for less than six months, two between six months and a year, nine between one and three years, seven between three and five years and five more than five years. As a group, they had few 'unusual' distinguishing features other than that no less than 15 of the 26 were described by their social workers as 'disturbed' to some degree. Approximately equal numbers had been admitted with brothers and sisters or alone and at the study start, ten were subject to care orders, and in a further seven the local authority had assumed parental rights and duties. In the year prior to the research just less than half (11) had at least monthly contact with one or both parents and at the study start approximately half were placed in foster homes, whilst two were home on trial. Twenty four of these 26 children remained in care during the study year.

Of the 29 children aged between 11 and 16 years, 19 were boys. Most (25) had been in care for at least a year, 12 for over five years. Two children were classified severely educationally sub-normal, another had difficulties related to his spasticity. In 17 of the 29 cases, the children were said to present behaviour difficulties. A third had been admitted to care with brothers or sisters and by the study start, 20 of the 29 were subject to care orders or the local authority had assumed parental rights and duties with respect to them. Eight of these youngsters had no contact with either parent in the year prior to the research, some none for many years, and ten had at least monthly contact. In contrast to younger children in this sub-sample, most (19) were in some type of residential care. Twenty six of the 29 remained in care throughout the study period.

Sixteen children comprised the final sub-grouping aged 16+ years with equal numbers of boys and girls. The majority (13) had already been in care for more than a year, eight for more than three years. Two children were severely mentally handicapped, one was classified as educationally sub-normal and six of the 16 children were described as presenting behaviour problems. Very few (3) had been admitted with brothers and sisters and at the study start 12 of the 16 were subject to some form of compulsory care. Five had had no contact with a parent for at least a year. At the time of their inclusion in the study, eight of these young people were in lodgings, bed-sitters or hostels, whilst three were in borstals. Most (13) reached the age of 18 during the study and left care, three remaining throughout.

Before concluding this chapter, attention is drawn to two more general points emerging from the above description. First, in accordance with the research design, there is little to indicate that as a group the the sample children were atypical of the children in care population as a whole. Hopefully, then, they provided us with access to a broad spread of decision-making patterns. Secondly whilst the purpose of this chapter has been to depict the setting and describe the characters on whom this research was based, rather than to provide study findings, it may nonetheless be significant to note the difference in rates of discharge from care between the two sub-samples: whilst eight of the 22 children under five in the into care sample remained in care throughout the year's study period, 22 of the 29 in care sample children did so. Similarly whilst only six of the 18 into care 5 to 11 year-olds remained in care, 24 of the corresponding 26 in care cases did so. In the older age range, the differences are less dramatic but nonetheless marked: for example of the 45 into care 11-16 year olds, 27 remained in care, whilst 26 of the 29 in care 11-16 year olds remained. Since the essential difference between these two sub-samples was the length of time the children had spent in care, it would certainly seem that as the length of time a child spends in care increases, the corresponding probability of returning home decreases (see also Rowe and Lambert, 1973 and Millham, *et al.*, forthcoming). This again suggests the importance of examining not only child and family characteristics, but also what happens once a child is in care.

Summary

The aim of the research design was to yield a selection of areas and children's cases which would serve as entry points to the process of social work decision-making and planning in child care. On the basis of the information provided in this chapter, we conclude that the research design was successful in generating a broad range of settings and individuals on which our study could be based. Having outlined the basic characteristics of the areas, social workers and children participating in the study, we adopt a thematic approach in the next six chapters concerned more specifically with the study findings.

CHAPTER THREE
Children's Care Careers

It was apparent from our preliminary work that courses of action taken in the early part of a child's career in care affected, and indeed restricted, the range of options and decisions possible at later stages of planning. Whilst this is perhaps self-evident, it impressed on us that a factor affecting length of time in care might well be the circumstances of the child's admission and the manner in which it was originally handled. This chapter begins by describing admission types and continues by exploring the link between different admission types and length of time in care.

Admission types

The fieldwork period left the strong, if crude impression that a distinction existed in terms of how young children and adolescents were dealt with in care. For this reason the 114 admissions and re-admissions during the study period were first classified according to age, under or over 11 years, at the time of admission. Ninety-five children were involved, the 85 cases of the into care sample and ten from the in care sample, the latter being included since they were admitted to care no more than eight weeks prior to the study start and in this sense, had more in common with the into care sample. Having so grouped the admissions, it became immediately apparent that whilst, in the main, behaviour difficulties characterised the group of older children, the younger age category comprised children admitted to care for widely differing types of reason.

Social workers had, of course, been asked the question 'Why was this child admitted to care?' Their very lengthy replies were in sharp contrast to the official categories of the annual statistical returns, tending to take the form of accounts of family situations and histories whose individuality was always stressed. From these replies it was certainly possible to identify a number of child and family characteristics in

26

common. However overall such characteristics indicated the sorts of circumstances in which a child is considered a likely candidate for care. The nature of the admission or why the admission actually occurred is left unexplained.

By widening the analysis of social workers' replies on all admissions to include the more general purpose they ascribed to admission, it was possible to identify three quite distinct themes. These themes were: the need to intervene in the family and rescue the child, offering a service to the family by temporarily relieving the family of the child, and finally the 'problem' behaviour of certain children and the need in some way to control it.

The 114 admissions were then grouped according to which of these themes, if any, was appropriate. Data about the children involved and what social workers thought was likely to happen to them were then added. Tables A3:1 to 4 in the Appendix detail these results. What became apparent was that it was possible to identify groups of cases, characterised not simply by distinguishing features of children and/or families but also by purpose of admission and anticipated length of time in care. Since the identifying data referred to circumstances at the time of admission, we have referred to each group of cases as an admission type. Table 3:1 outlines the distribution of the admission types — child behaviour, rescue from the family and service to the family — across the 114 admissions. We can be relatively confident in ascribing all but seven of the admissions to an admission type. Arguably two of these seven cases should not have been included in the sample since they involved children placed by their parents with the local authority for adoption. The remaining five admissions contained elements of at least two admission-types and were not so readily classifiable.

Table 3.1
The 114 admissions: distribution by admission type

Admission type	No.	%
Child behaviour	45	40
Rescue from the family	34	30
Service to the family	28	24
Other	7	6
Total	**114**	**100**

'Child behaviour' admissions (n = 45)

This type of admission accounted for 40 per cent of the total admissions in the study period. The children involved were a disparate group in many respects but were all adolescents (over the age of 11) and predominantly male. In common their social workers' accounts of the reasons for their entry to care emphasised the child's behaviour. A wide range of behaviour was reported: for example, the difficulties of below average intelligence adolescents, adolescent rebellion within the home, school attendance problems, cultural conflicts between ethnic minority parents and their children and anti-social behaviour of a criminal nature.

Whilst it was the child's behaviour which was identified as creating the need for care, the behaviour had nonetheless been occurring for some time prior to entry to care. It appeared to us, then, to offer only a partial explanation of why admission took place at a particular time. On the assumption that such admissions occur when the child's behaviour is defined by the social services department as problematic, we examined the events and exchanges preceding entry to care. The significance of the influence, and indeed power, of other agencies thus became apparent and was identified as operating in two distinct ways.

First in approximately two-thirds of the admissions, it was evident that the child's parents or school, for example, had been demanding that the social services department 'should be doing something' about a child. In other words, the young person's behaviour was being identified as problematic and in need of control by other agencies or individuals in contact with him. Such admissions were generally preceded by an act of the young person, not itself of particular note but which, by cumulative effect, heightened the concern of these parties. In turn, this served to renew their pressure on the social worker to take some action. The process is illustrated by the following case:

> Tom was a 13-year-old-boy from a family described by the social worker as 'a well-known problem family'. For many years he had been the subject of discussion between the social services and education departments because of his poor school attendance.
>
> According to the social worker, 'I have never been unduly concerned — it's a family we keep an eye on but really they function very well in their own way. The problem is the way we — society — think people should behave. It comes down to values in the end and I don't feel just because they (the family) don't conform to every petty

social norm that that is a reason for putting the kid away'. He reported, on the other hand, that the boy's school and the education department advocated his removal from home and had done so for several years.

In an attempt to resolve these difficulties, it had been mutually agreed that the social worker, rather than the educational welfare officer, would attempt to ensure the boy's attendance. This was agreed at a meeting prior to the start of a school year and the social worker did succeed in securing the boy's attendance in the short-term. As soon as his attendance became irregular again, the school contacted the social worker and he responded by suggesting and eventually obtaining the boy's mother's consent to voluntary care.

The social worker informed us that his own view had not changed but he felt that he had to accede to the school's viewpoint. Asked why the boy had been admitted to care he replied. 'Because of his school attendance — it was getting to the stage that the school were ringing me up every day and I think to be honest when he was there, which wasn't often, they made life so uncomfortable for him, that they were really driving him away. I had to do something'.

In some cases an act of a young person resulted in a further party becoming involved and they, too, might demand that something should be done. The effect of such a widening of concern appeared to reduce the confidence of social workers in resisting admission. In this respect, the introduction of police involvement was especially significant. For example we found that when the police became involved in a case, social workers rarely objected to them pressing criminal charges and, indeed would recommend a care order at a subsequent court hearing. Parents, too, could be highly influential. If they began to complain of the child when concern was already being expressed by professional agencies, the child's admission invariably followed.

The distinctive feature of these admissions was that the demands of the other agencies or individuals had the effect of exerting pressure on social services staff 'to do something'. Social services personnel, however, did not always share their definition of the problem or their view of how it should be tackled. The resulting admission can therefore be seen as a form of response to the efforts of other agencies to relieve themselves of the problem.

In the remaining third of admissions based on the child's behaviour, the social worker had already defined the child's behaviour as a problem and consideration was being given to how to deal with it. In such cases, however, admission did not commonly occur until such time as another agency became involved and expressed concern. Here, the knowledge and concern of other agencies were used to support the act of admission. For example, it was noted that if the police initiated criminal prosecution, the social worker would recommend a care order despite the fact that the offence was trivial and only the first the child was known to have committed. In such cases, social workers openly admitted that they were using the opportunity provided by criminal proceedings, rather than risking an unsuccessful approach to the court on other grounds. Similarly, it was noted that care was often negotiated with the education department. Here for instance, when it became known that a child causing concern to the social services department was also a poor attender at school, agreement was reached that the education department would initiate care proceedings on the basis of school attendance and the social worker would recommend a care order.

However, whether, as in these admissions, the role of other agencies was that of supplying evidence of the shared concern, or that of applying pressure on social services, it was clear that those dealing with the case did not necessarily consider admission to care as an appropriate response. In questioning social workers about the *purpose* of admitting a child to care under the above circumstances, the control element of care became evident and social workers were vague, if not openly pessimistic about what care might offer. From their point of view, admission to care was an option in a fairly limited repertoire of responses to young people in trouble. These points are illustrated in the following replies by social workers:

> I am not sure really — I just felt we had to do something — the situation was doing nobody any good. But what can we do? I don't know — often at the end of these cases you say to yourself — 'What have we done . . . .? You know it's often worse after we've been in'.

and

> It's difficult to say — you can never say if it will work, far less how. To some youngsters it's the shock and that does the trick. Sometimes it acts as a breathing space and that's all that's required. You just don't know — it comes to the point where you have to step in — society, I suppose, expects it.

30 Although 40 per cent of the admissions in the study period were portrayed as occurring because of adolescent behaviour difficulties, this represents an incomplete picture of the processes leading to admission to care. Social workers' often negative assessment of the value of care in these circumstances and, on the other hand, the pressure to be seen 'to be doing something' about a clearly difficult situation, must also be taken into account. An alternative way of viewing the admission to care of youngsters such as these is as a resolution of the pressure 'to do something'. The dilemma of what that might achieve appears often to be left on one side at this stage.

'Rescue from the family' admissions (n = 34)

This type of admission accounted for 30 per cent of the overall admissions in the study period. Children of all ages were involved but the majority of admissions (31) involved children under the age of 11 years. Social workers stated 'risk to the child' as the underlying reason for these admissions and in admitting the child to care, social workers were, by their intervention, rescuing the child from the family.

From our interviews with social workers, it was apparent that 'risk to the child' could take many forms: possible, as well as actual, physical abuse, and neglect, both physical and emotional. These categories however, disguise the difficulties inherent in establishing that circumstances in an individual case constitute risk and that a child's removal from home may be necessary. Detailed examination of events preceding admission indicate that this is a process which can be both anxiety-provoking and time-consuming.

In 14 of the 34 admissions there had been longstanding concern about the care the child was receiving at home and admission was preceded by what, at first sight, might appear a trivial incident but was perceived by social workers as forming part of an emerging pattern of risk. Several of the children involved had previously been in care on more than one occasion and, in general, the question of their removal from home had been under consideration for some time prior to admission. The incident preceding their entry to care provided both an opportunity to remove the child and substantive evidence in the preparation of the case for court. A typical comment made in relation to these admissions was: 'it's been a question of waiting for the right moment'.

In such cases, it was considered that the existence of 'risk' had already been established; in the remaining 20 cases, the *potential* for 'risk' prompted admission. Here 'others' were defining the child as being at risk and social services responded to this 'to be on the safe side'. In eight of these 20 admissions, for example, the admission was preceded by several requests by the child's parents that 'something be done' and occurred at the point where the child was abandoned or the parents reported or threatened non-accidental injury to the child. In a similar number of cases, intervention and the child's removal from the family was initiated by another agency, particularly the police. Where the police took a place of safety order and initiated care proceedings, the social services recommended a care order, acknowledging to us that while, in their opinion, the home situation had not changed, 'it's better to be safe than sorry'.

With few exceptions, the cases involved in admissions based on the notion of rescue from the family were already known to the social services department and indeed most were registered cases. They were nonetheless described as 'emergency' admissions. To some extent this description may reflect the anxiety felt by social workers at having to consider a child's removal from home and indeed such admissions were generally characterised by lack of certainty about the child's future.

This anxiety was also evident in social workers' replies to being asked about the purpose of care. Whilst occasionally references were made to the 'safety of the child', the commonly used phrases were 'there was no alternative' and 'we had no choice'. Though the social work profession is often accused of 'child snatching', it was interesting to note that the social workers here appeared to admit children to care with reluctance, and indeed were often apologetic about having taken such action. They said for example:

> We don't like taking children into care and we try to avoid it where at all possible.

> Care is always the last step.

> It's not something we like doing but it's sometimes inevitable.

Comments such as these, implying both a general reluctance to take the step of admitting to care and the eventual inevitability of such a course of action in individual cases, suggest that the act of admission may represent a contradiction in terms for social workers. How they deal with this contradiction in subsequent stages of the care process may well have implications for the child.

'Service to the family' admissions (n = 28)

These admissions accounted for 24 per cent of all admissions in the study period and numerically they formed the smallest group. As with the previous group, children of all ages were involved but only four were over the age of 11 years. The notion of service to the family underlay admissions where the situation referred to the social services department represented a family crisis, which was expected to be only temporary. Examples of such situations are when a parent was admitted to hospital, and when parents, or more commonly a mother and her cohabitee, separated and new accommodation had to be found. Occasionally, too, children were admitted to care on the basis of an agreement between the social services department and the parent in a single parent family that care could be used for temporary relief. In other words, then, service to the family admissions occurred on the understanding that the child's separation from the family represented a brief interruption to family life, not a substitute for it.

In 18 of these 28 admissions, it was the family who approached the department, specifially requesting that their child, or more often their children, be admitted to care. We noted that admission did not always automatically follow but that alternative arrangements or services, such as a residential family aide would first be suggested by the social worker. The parents, nonetheless, persisted in seeking care. In a few cases, the route to care took the form of a family approaching the department with a problem and making a more general request for help. The social worker again suggested a range of alternatives, only one of which was the child's admission to care. Having been advised to return home and consider these options, the family returned to the department seeking care. Two points are worth making here. First, the parents viewed care positively and as a service to the family and secondly, as was noted with the two other types of admission, social workers approached the question of admission with hesitation and reluctance.

Interestingly, whilst this type of admission tended to occur at the request of parents, few of the cases involved were subject to ongoing social work contact and indeed several were entirely unknown to the social services department prior to the application for care. Despite this, and the fact that the request for care stemmed from some form of crisis, the resulting admissions, were described as 'planned'. It appeared that, having eventually agreed to the child entering care and feeling no great anxiety about the long-term future, the social worker involved did not

In Care

feel under undue pressure in organising how admission should occur. In describing the purpose of such admissions social workers tended to make statements such as 'admission was in the interest of the family' or 'admission was what the parents wanted'.

Length of time in care

These three groups emerged in the first place from analysis of information collected at the time of admission to care. By following the care careers of the individual children involved in each of the three groups over the next year, it became apparent that patterns of care duration corresponded with each admission type. Table 3:2 sets out by admission type, the number of cases which continued through the study period and those which left care during it, showing a highly significant relationship between admission type and length of time in care.

In other words, children entering care as a service to the family are likely to remain in care for less time than children admitted to care for other reasons. From Table 3:2, it would appear that children entering care as rescue from the family or child behaviour admissions have similar chances of leaving or remaining in care. However, this is not to suggest that both groups are likely to remain in care for similar lengths of time. It should be remembered, for example, that child behaviour admissions tended to involve older children and as such the length of time such children might spend in care was unlikely to exceed five years.

The differing rates of discharge from care of each of the admission types is more clearly depicted in Table 3.3. This table points out that

Table 3.2
The Into-care Group: type of admission to care and duration

Type of admission	In care a year later		Terminating within the year		Total	
	n	%	n	%		
Child behaviour	29	64	16	36	**45**	**100**
Rescue from the family	20	59	14	41	**34**	**100**
Service to the family	4	14	24	86	**28**	**100**
Other	3	43	4	57	**7**	**100**
Total	**56**	**49**	**58**	**51**	**114**	**100**

Table 3.3
The Into-care Group: rates of discharge from care according to type of admission

Duration in care	Child behaviour		Rescue from the family		Service to the family		Three groups combined	
	n	%	n	%	n	%	n	%
Less than 1 week	1		2		5		8	
Between 1-2 weeks	1		1		6		8	
Between 2 weeks-1 month	2		4		6		12	
Total under 1 month	4	9	7	20	17	60	28	24
Between 1-3 months	6		5		5		16	
Between 3-6 months	4		1		2		7	
Total between 1-6 months	10	22	6	17	7	25	23	20
Total under 6 months	14	31	13	38	24	85	51	43
Total in sample	**45**	**100**	**34**	**100**	**28**	**100**	**107**	**100**

when looking at all admissions the rate of leaving care decreases as time progresses, with almost half the admissions terminating within the first six months. Between groups, however, there were marked contrasts.

On the basis, then, that length of time in care was at least in part related to type of admission, we used our background information on the remaining 90 cases of the in-care group to apply the same classification. Surprisingly, perhaps, we found that the three admission types again applied. Table 3:4 sets out the in-care group according to admission type and length of time already in care at the study start.

None of these 90 cases had been in care for less than six months at the study start, and it would therefore appear from our sample that the population of children in care over six months is likely to be dominated by admissions based on the notion of rescuing the child from the family. Moreover, while the table suggests that most child behaviour admissions spend between one and three years in care, it is clear that admissions based on rescue from service to the family may remain in care for quite considerable periods of time. In the case of service to the family admissions, this is rather suprising since social workers generally expected such cases to return home quickly. It would therefore appear that the small proportion of service to the family admissions who do not leave quickly remain and linger in care for lengthy spells.

In Care

Table 3.4
The In Care Group: type of admission and length of time in care at study start

Length of time in care at study start	Child behaviour		Rescue from the family		Service to family		Other		Total	
	n	%	n	%	n	%	n	%	n	%
6 mths-year	3		7		6		–		16	18
1-2 years	7		5		3		1		16	18
2-3 years	6		9		1		–		16	18
3-4 years	2		8		3		–		13	15
4-5 years	3		2		3		–		8	8
5-10 years	–		7		5		1		13	15
10-15 years	–		2		2		–		4	4
Over 15 years	–		–		3		1		4	4
Total	**21**	**23**	**40**	**45**	**26**	**29**	**3**	**3**	**90**	**100**

These figures, of course, provide only a very rough guide: the children involved entered care over a time-span of over 15 years, a period of changing emphases in social work and we have no knowledge of the size of the cohorts of children who entered care at the same time but subsequently left. Nonetheless certain 'risk' categories are identifiable.

The data in Table 3:5 suggest that the rate of leaving care further reduces after five years in care, and indeed four of the five discharges occurring after more than four years in care did so because the child had reached the age of 18. In terms of type of admission, this table further indicates the higher rate of discharge from care of the child behaviour group, otherwise the numerically smallest group. On the other hand, rescue from the family admissions, numerically the largest group, show a relatively lower rate of discharge from care. Although, then, these three admission types were initially used to describe the 114 admissions in the study period, admission type does appear to be of some significance to length of time in care. For this reason we use the same categorisation for all the study cases in subsequent stages of the report when considering aspects of children's careers in care and social work decision making in more detail.

Table 3.5
The In Care Group: those leaving care in study period according to length of time in care at study start

Length of time in care at	Child behaviour		Rescue from the family		Service to family		Other		Total	
	n	%	n	%	n	%	n	%	n	%
6 months-1 year	–		2		1		–		3	13
1-2 years	2		1		1		–		4	17
2-3 years	2		1		–		–		3	13
3-4 years	2		3		3		–		8	35
4-5 years	2		–		–		–		2	9
5-10 years	–		7		5		1		13	15
10-15 years	–		–		–		–		0	0
Over 15 years	–		–		2		–		2	9
Total leaving care	8		7		8		–		23	100
Total excluding those leaving on account of age	5	24	6	15	5	19	–		16	18

Summary

The topic of admission to care was included in the study since it was suggested that what occurred at the point of admission could largely determine a child's future career in care. In this chapter, three admission types have been identified, each implying a different client focus. In 'service to the family' admissions, emphasis was on the family and its continuance; in 'rescue from the family' admissions, emphasis was on the child, with the child's future a matter of uncertainty; and 'child behaviour' admissions, where emphasis was on control of the child. On the basis of looking at admissions to care during the study period, it appeared that service to the family admissions tend to leave care much more rapidly than other admissions, 85 per cent leaving within the first six months. By applying the same classification to the cases already in care at the study start, it did however appear that service to the family admissions, who did not leave care within six months, might remain in care for a considerable period of time. Child behaviour admissions, on the other hand, were unlikely to leave care within six months of admission but did not appear to remain more than five years. A different pattern again emerges with admissions based on the notion of rescue from the family: whilst almost 40 per cent of the new admissions of this type left care within six months of entry to care, 45 per cent of all children in care for over six months were of this type. During the study period 15 per cent of these left care, all within five years of admission though not necessarily by returning to their families.

CHAPTER FOUR
Deciding to Admit to Care

The significance of the event of admission to care for the various parties involved — the child, the parent and indeed the social services department — was recognised by most of the authorities participating in the study, and in each a large section of the departmental procedure manual was devoted to this topic. Details varied from authority to authority but took an essentially similar form. The basic requirements for admission were set out, such as the forms it was necessary to complete and who were required to be contacted. Basically, *procedures* were described although, occasionally, guidance on the professional aspect of admission was offered, for example, the desirability of pre-placement visits might be stressed. Overall, however, it was recognised that flexibility was necessary and admission could not be subject to a standardised code of prescriptions. Significantly for us, such procedures and guidelines did not endeavour to stipulate, beyond the official legislative categories, under what circumstances a child should be admitted to care or how that decision should be reached. The purpose of this chapter is to describe how and by whom the decision to admit to care is taken. Like the previous chapter it is based primarily on the 114 new admissions during the study period.

The act of admission to care is not a unitary event. As Hilgendorf (1981) has pointed out 'it is a process which may take place over a long period and involve many individuals, professional groups and agencies'. In the previous chapter we have indicated the influence, and indeed power, of such agencies. Admission to care is also a multi-stage operation which involves not one but a number of decisions each of which may impact on the other. For example, the question of the legislation under which admission might occur, and where the child is to be placed must also be given consideration before admission can occur. In addition, during analysis of this part of our data, it became evident that the pattern of parent-child contact established at the time of admission to care could be significant to the child's future. The consideration given to each of these questions as the child enters care is dealt with here according to the different admission types.

Child behaviour admissions (n = 45)

Who takes the decision to admit to care?

Over 70 per cent of the children concerned in these admissions were already known to the social services department prior to their being admitted to local authority care. Nonetheless in eight cases (more than 15 per cent), social workers maintained that the department had not been party to the admission decision. Each of these cases had involved the court making a care order, generally in criminal proceedings. In three instances the social services department had not participated in the decision, because, due to an administrative oversight, they had not been informed of the proceedings. In the remaining five cases, the departments were aware of and involved in the proceedings to the extent that a social worker had submitted a background report to the court. However, the writers of these reports had made no recommendation to the court because, whilst individually they all felt admission to be inappropriate in the circumstances, they nonetheless anticipated this was what the court would decide. Not wishing to associate themselves with such an outcome, they had left their reports 'open'.

However in the vast majority of cases, the decision to admit to care was stated as the decision of the social services department and, in general, some form of discussion was said to have taken place between the social worker dealing with the case and at least one more senior member of staff. Asked who was involved in the decision to admit, typical social worker replies were as follows:

> My team leader and myself — I raised it and I think we both agreed that this is what should happen.

> I had a word with my team leader about the situation — I think we jointly agreed to go for a care order.

Only two social workers maintained that they had taken the decision to admit a study child to care without specifically discussing it with a more senior colleague, both implying that this was unusual. Typically, then, child behaviour admissions were preceded by some form of discussion within the social services department, these discussions being described by the social worker concerned as informal.

40   Two particular phenomena appeared to contribute to the fact that

these admissions were generally discussed prior to the child's entry. First, although we found no evidence of it in official departmental policy, we were struck by the extent to which social workers felt it was inappropriate to admit an older child to care. They felt this was something to be regretted, if not avoided. The notion of admitting a child of this age to *voluntary care* was particularly alien and, as was mentioned in the previous chapter, taking action would be delayed until such time as it was possible to organise admission to compulsory care. Likewise we noted that few older children were admitted to care via care proceedings on the grounds that their development was being avoidably impaired, school attendance grounds or criminal proceedings being preferred. Between areas, there were variations in the extent to which the inappropriateness of care to the older child functioned as an operational principle. Overall, however, such was the strength of feeling about this that case holders tended to keep their team leaders closely acquainted with those cases where care was a possiblity.

Secondly the influence or pressure exerted by other agencies lends political overtones to the situation where there is a possibility of an older child being admitted to care. This was most conspicuous in relation to the court: no less than 11 of the 27 social workers submitting reports to the court commented that in writing these reports they were influenced by the almost certain knowledge that 'the court was unlikely to wear anything other than a care order'. The same situation applied in relation to the education services and the police, main grade social workers expressing a high degree of ambivalence towards both. On the one hand, social workers resented the pressure they felt other agencies exerted on them to admit a child to care, and on the other recognised their own inability to refuse a referral. Satyamurti (1981) has described this situation as a system of 'asymmetrical exchange' in which certain parties to the interaction are in a more favourable position than others. Here, social workers were aware of the need to maintain a minimal balance in relationships with other professional agencies both at the individual and departmental levels. Where they felt under pressure from other agencies to follow certain paths, they tended to consult higher agency personnel. However, although there was likely to be discussion prior to such a decision, this is not to deny that, within social services departments, social workers are key decision makers. Other members of staff were certainly party to the decision to admit to care, but this was largely an involvement by association, it being social workers who actually determined whether or not a child entered care. Social workers reported, for instance, that they would use the opportunity provided by criminal proceedings to achieve admission when they anticipated that voluntary admission would not be favoured within the department. For example, in referring to the recent admission of a 15-year-old, the social worker said:

> I have spoken to my senior about Jean several times. We talked about trying to get her a place in (specialised form of residential care) but I realised (team leader) wasn't all that keen so when the shoplifting thing came up, I thought I might as well try it this way.

Social workers also negotiated with parents to achieve admission. For example, when both social workers and parent favoured admission but it was anticipated that voluntary admission would be rejected within the agency, social workers would suggest that the parents either write to the department or approach the police stating the child to be beyond their control. This occurred in four study cases, the social workers concerned reporting that given this situation there was no alternative other than to initiate care proceedings. The case of Ben illustrates particularly well the extent to which social workers may retain residual power, enabling them to manipulate situations as they deem appropriate.

> Ben was admitted to care twice during the study period. Prior to the first occasion, both his mother and school claimed that they could do nothing with him, and eventually he was admitted to care. Following assessment, the education department agreed to place him in a residential special school and Ben was discharged from care on the understanding that he should return to his mother during the school holidays. When this time came, his mother accepted him but with some reluctance and frequently contacted the social worker complaining of his behaviour. According to the social worker. 'We resisted taking him into care but felt we would probably have to for the long summer holidays'.
>
> However, Ben's mother was distraught and asked for his removal. The social worker's team leader felt nothing would be achieved by short-term care and that the social worker should attempt to keep the boy at home until the start of term again. Nonetheless Ben's mother was persistent and according to the social worker, 'I suggested that the only thing I thought she could do was to write to the department or the police stating that she couldn't control him'. When I left she had calmed down a bit but Ben still hadn't come home. The next morning I discovered he had come back after midnight,

drunk — mother had taken him straight to the police station stating 'he is yours, I can't stand this any more and marched out'. The police obtained a place of safety order on Ben and initiated care proceedings on the grounds that he was beyond parental control. The social worker then recommended, and the court made, a care order.

As many of the children involved in child behaviour admissions were admitted to observation and assessment centres prior to the making of a full care order, we anticipated that assessment centre staff and assessment case conferences would play a significant role in deciding to admit to care. In our experience, this was the case only when the courts requested an assessment centre report, that is for six of the 24 children initially placed in observation and assessment centres. More commonly full case conferences did not take place until some time after the making of a care order and although social workers did tend to consult centre staff about the child's admission to care, this was on an informal basis and the initiative for admission was retained by fieldwork staff.

Our data to date point up the complex nature of the decision to admit to care. In the previous chapter we highlighted the important role played by other professional agencies and indeed parents. Here we have indicated the nature of the discussions which take place within the social services department prior to care. Despite the strategic importance of other individuals and agencies a key figure in the decision to admit — although subject to many constraints — is nonetheless the social worker holding the case.

Choice of legal status

It should not be assumed because of the order of presentation here that decisions about legal status are necessarily taken after the decision to admit. In practice this is rarely the case. Social workers tend not to address the issue of legal status explicitly in the sense of seeing it as a discrete decision they have to take. More commonly the features which influence choice of status are seen as integral characteristics of the presenting problem. The selection of appropriate legal status is, therefore, inextricably bound up with the implicit attitudes and conditions governing entry to care and, as such, may determine whether or not admission occurs. Determination of the legal status under which a child enters care therefore emerges from the inter-play of some apparently quite unrelated factors, and it is unlikely that who ultimately makes the decision about legal status can be separated from who makes the decision about admission. Again, the social worker is in a key position.

Since the purpose underlying the majority of these child behaviour admissions was the need to 'control' the young person, control, not surprisingly, was the feature most frequently referred to in the selection of the legislation under which the admission would occur. Given the importance ascribed to the notion of 'control' it is perhaps equally unsurprising that there was little evidence of social workers routinely seeking the views of young people about their admission. Social workers did, however, have views of the extent to which a young person would be 'co-operative' and this could influence the degree of importance placed on the control element. For example, a young person who it was felt recognised the disruptive nature of his behaviour and wished to change it was more likely to be considered for voluntary care than one who did not.

However the need for control was not the only consideration in determining legal status. Also important in this context, and already referred to, was the notion that it was inappropriate to admit older children to voluntary care. Thus, even although in a number of cases the child's family requested admission and admission could therefore have been voluntary, such a request was refused. In the same cases, if criminal proceedings later followed, or care proceedings were brought on the basis of the parents stating that the child was beyond their control, the social services recommended a care order. The objective here was to ensure that if the child was to be admitted to care, control was relatively assured. In a couple of cases the procedure went wrong and the court did not make a care order. Ironically too, in a further two cases voluntary care was arranged because, despite the fact that court proceedings were initiated, the solicitor appointed on behalf of a child argued that since both parents and social worker favoured care, there was no need for court involvement.

However not all child behaviour admissions were admitted to compulsory care and in this respect it is interesting to note the concern expressed by several social workers about the number of young people approaching the department seeking care. In certain instances this was said to reflect a genuine breakdown in family relationships and ultimately the child concerned was admitted to care without the parents signing the consent to admission forms. This step was justified by social workers who stated: 'control wasn't really essential here' and 'we could have gone to court but that would have been traumatic for everyone'.

In other cases social workers felt that underlying the young person's request for care was the belief that care offered better material standards than those available at home. Requests such as these were generally refused in the first place, not because the social worker was unsympathetic to the individual youngster but because it was considered 'wrong to admit adolescents to voluntary care'. Social workers explained that the voluntary admission of two such study cases was appropriate since entry to care permitted these children to continue with an educational course. Here the presenting problem had been translated in such a way that the need for the control element was less apparent. Other youngsters who requested admission to care were described as 'having worked the system': having realised that requesting their own admission was unlikely to be successful they ensured that appearance before court for school attendance or offences and entered care by that route.

Choice of placement

In theory, two decisions are involved in deciding where to place a child on admission to care: what type of placement is to be chosen and within type, what actual placement is to be selected. In practice, the existence of assumptions about the appropriateness of certain types of placement meant that the element of choice was minimalised and the distinction between decisions about type of placement and decisions about actual placement was rarely explicit.

Type of placement

The vast majority, (almost 80 per cent) of child behaviour admissions were placed on admission in residential care. Nonetheless, the high proportion so placed was not a reflection of social workers' preference for this form of care. Indeed many were openly critical of the range of provision of residential care for adolescents and of the quality of care it offered. In this context, adjectives such as 'pathetic' and 'abysmal' were often used. Nothwithstanding this, however, it was quite clear that choice of *type* of placement was governed by the assumption that adolescents, (and child behaviour admissions tended to involve adolescents), are placed in residential care. For example, almost half the child behaviour admissions resulted in placements in observation and assessment centres and explaining the reasons for this, social workers described it as 'routine' or 'standard' practice. Similar comments were made of placement in community homes: 'it's where we always place adolescent girls' and 'that's where we generally place youngsters of this age'. Overwhelmingly then, there was a tendency to equate adolescent care with residential provision.

In several of the remaining admissions (approximately 20 per cent), the child's placement tended to pre-date entry to care, foster homes and lodging type accommodation being involved. At the time of admission, these placements were either felt suitable for the child to remain in or indeed, the sole purpose of admission had been to allow the child to continue in the placement. In these, then, selection of placement type was already partially determined. In only three of the remaining cases had the type of accommodation been specifically chosen: a hostel was specifically sought for a boy over 16 at the time of admission and the low proportion of children in foster care was not a reflection of foster homes being sought and not provided but of the fact that fostering was not considered for the majority of child behaviour admissions.

Actual placement Although many child behaviour admissions resulted in placements in observation and assessment centres, there was little evidence to suggest that the purpose of the placements was assessment of the child. Indeed many of the children concerned were already well known to the social workers and even prior to admission had been the subject of frequent discussions with other agencies. The many purposes placement in such establishments may serve is demonstrated in the following social worker comments:

> No one could think of anything else sufficiently controlling . . . he is a known absconder. Nothing else has the same security.

> It was an emergency. I had to get him a bed somewhere. They *(observation and assessment centre staff)* usually oblige with a bed, anyway.

> I imagine this is going to be a CHE case and you need an assessment report for that — they just won't consider you without it.

> I've been arguing with education for a month now but they won't give him a place. If only they *(observation and assessment staff)* agree with me, their opinion is much more highly regarded than mine.

Social workers' replies in relation to other residential placements indicated that ideally they considered a 'treatment' approach to be appropriate. For example:

> What he needs is an environment where he is helped to see beyond what his own experience has taught him. . . and it needs to be done quickly.

> She is not being allowed to grow at home and she is rebelling against that. She needs a place to grow and help in coming to terms with her approaching adulthood.

Social workers nonetheless felt that the provision available did not match what was required and that, in reality, there was little choice other than that of a community home or a community school. The former were considered to be limited in scope and whilst social workers appreciated that, in some instances, the head of the home was enthusiastic to adopt innovative approaches to children, their experience suggested that, in practice, those who daily dealt with the young people rarely had the skills, and sometimes not the inclination, to implement them. On the other hand, they described community schools as 'regimes' and indicated what they felt was their 'total inappropriateness' to the needs of many young people.

In other words the range of options both of type and of actual placement was narrowly defined by social workers. Like foster placements, the allocation of residential placements was commonly the responsibility of a special member of staff or section and the typical response to questions about choice of placement was 'there was no choice — you have to take what you can get'. The only real exception to this was where children had been placed in an observation and assessment centre. Here, although social workers did not necessarily agree with the recommendation of the assessment case conference, they rarely objected to it. Since observation and assessment centre staff tend to assume, as part of their overall responsibilities, the role of negotiating a child's entry to a recommended placement, the extensive use of observation and assessment centres may serve the purpose of enabling social workers to feel that they are not entirely responsible for taking a decision which, by their definition, is not satisfactory.

Departmentally, then, and in so far as child behaviour admissions were concerned, social workers appeared to have considerable scope to influence decisions about the child's entry to care. Although their influence was at times constrained by organisational factors, including resources, it was also apparent that at times they voluntarily relinquished their ability to influence. This was most conspicuous in decisions which social workers felt were based on inappropriate principles, contrary to their own professional judgement. The control element underlying these child behaviour admissions was one such principle often deemed inappropriate by social workers, and could represent for them an ideological conflict. Given that they may deal with that conflict at the time of admission by relinquishing their influence raises the question of the implications this may also have for the child post-entry to care. This point is taken up later in the report when what happens after entry to care is discussed.

Decisions about parent-child contact

Although social workers were not specifically questioned about parent-child contact at the time of admission, we noted that they rarely reported decisions about this to us. Likewise, in outlining the manner in which placement decisions had been reached, social workers rarely made mention of the implications of their decisions for parent-child contact.

This is not to say that decisions on this matter are not taken, but that they are rarely taken explicitly (see also Millham *et al*, forthcoming). The children involved here were older children and their age and placement impinged on the nature of decisions about contact with their families. In the first place, contact for these children generally meant the young person visiting parents rather than vice versa, to some extent this being a reflection of the older child's capacity to travel without supervision. However it is also important to recognise that in the world of the adolescent, 'going home' is as much to do with contact with the area and peers as it is with parent and family. Therefore, the social worker had to consider the implications of contact with peers, when deciding about home visits. Peers, as opposed to the family, were often a source of concern to social workers and thus, decisions about contact with parents could be taken indirectly. Secondly the vast majority of these admissions resulted in placement in residential care where visits home form an important part of a system of rewards and punishment. However, although there was generally an early agreement between residential staff and social workers about the frequency of 'weekend leave', we did note that residential staff altered such arrangements without necessarily consulting the social worker. Whilst several social workers described this as a source of dissatisfaction, we nonetheless found that they rarely conveyed this to the residential staff concerned and appeared to be basically content to leave the matter to someone else.

In other words, the question of contact with parents and family readily became a secondary issue in these admissions and was influenced by the taking of decisions on other matters rather than as a decision *per se*. As such, decisions on parent-child contact may be described as decisions by default.

Rescue from the family admissions. (n = 34)

Who takes the decisions to admit to care?

Since the majority of children involved in rescue from the family admissions were already known to the department, and care was not entirely unanticipated, the decision to admit to care was generally one which evolved over time. According to social workers, the child's entry to care was preceded by departmental discussion but the form and significance of that discussion was seen to vary widely and, in general, was much less conspicuous than in child behaviour admissions. In only three instances did an inter-agency case conference take place prior to admission and more commonly, social workers replied as follows: 'I must have spoken to someone about it but I can't recall anything specific'.

Furthermore while departmental procedures required that admission to care be approved by senior agency officials, such as the team leader or area director, social workers saw this as 'a rubber stamping exercise'. They acknowledged that they might have spoken to their team leader but were insistent that they alone had taken the decision. Thus as far as social workers were concerned, the notion of seeking approval was not part of these discussions, whose purpose they otherwise described in the following manner:

> I did mention it to my team leader who knows the case, but it wasn't a formal decision between the two of us. It was just in conversation and I said 'This is what I am going to do if nothing else turns up'.

> I always talk to someone — my team leader or somebody — about admission to care — to sound out my feelings. But I wouldn't say they made the decision — not even with me. I couldn't call them responsible for it in any way.

49

In Care

In contrast to child behaviour admissions, then, the emerging picture is one which supports the view that frontline social workers determine who enters care. A few exceptions to this were, nonetheless, noted. For example, previously unknown cases of non-accidental injury tended to be referred to a more senior representative of the social services department and the decision to admit the child to care was influenced more by the referring agency and other professionals already acquainted with the case than the newly assigned social worker. Such cases were however, rare. We also noted that in some ongoing cases where the social worker acknowledged the need for intervention but the family were resistant to help, the team leader, area director and occasionally a representative of the authority's legal department became involved in establishing the department's legal authority to intervene. In these circumstances, social workers described those party to the discussion as full participants in the decision.

These were, however, exceptions and on the whole it was frontline social workers who determined who entered care. Furthermore although social workers often indicated that it was a no-choice decision which they took, it was clear that they were aware of the strategic position they occupied. As one social worker put it:

> I certainly have a great deal of influence. I can manipulate the situation if you like, choose what to relay and what not, select where I put the emphasis.

Choice of legal status

In rescue from the family admissions, the legislation under which the child is admitted to care may be particularly important: it has implications for the parents of the child and their involvement in planning for him or her and for the social services department, it may be necessary to reinforce their right to intervene in the family. Just over half (19) of the 34 children involved in these admissions entered care compulsorily.

Broadly speaking, the data here suggest that choice of legal status tends to be based on assumptions about what best befits certain types of situation. In general two criteria appear to be of particular importance, although they are not entirely independent: the parents' attitude to care, and the perceived need for some sort of control of the situation by the social services department. Thus, voluntary care was described as:

All that was necessary,

or

All that was required as the parents were in agreement . . .

Whereas of compulsory care, it was said:

It seemed that the time had come for us to have more control.

In rescue from the family admissions another factor was occasionally significant. Here the relative importance ascribed to the notion of parental co-operation, or as social workers put it: 'working with parents' could over-ride the more generally observed criteria. The variable treatment of non-accidental injury cases indicated the extent to which this could be encapsulated in a departmental view. In most areas, for example, it was automatic that cases such as these would be dealt with by initiating care proceedings in court. If there was any uncertainty about the legal basis for this, voluntary admission was resisted even though it might be requested by parents, in order to allow compulsory steps to be taken in the future.

Elsewhere, however, if the parents were willing to have the child admitted, voluntary admission was deemed preferable. In these departments, even when the parents were initially unwilling to contemplate admission, there was prolonged and intensive discussion with them in an effort to obtain their co-operation and consent and this occurred despite it being known that a legal basis for seeking a care order existed, and the prognosis for the child's future in the family was by no means certain.

The significance social workers ascribed to the idea of 'working with parents' was evident in a further respect. For example in a few study cases, social workers appeared to have little intention of admitting a child to compulsory care. However if action was taken by someone other than the case holder, such as the night duty officer or another agency, which facilitated a hearing in court, the social worker carrying the case was then prepared to continue the process and recommend a care order. In adopting this approach, social workers felt that they were not only obtaining 'some control' in the case but that tolerable relations with parents could still be maintained. The child's admission to compulsory care was thus made acceptable by the involvement of another individual or agency.

51

The question, therefore, of who decides the legal status under which such admissions occur is not simply answered. While the choices made are complex and bound up in the immediate nature of the admission, a considerable degree of influence is nonetheless held by the individual social worker holding the case. On occasions the legal issue over-shadowed the very question of admission and in these circumstances the opinion of a representative of the authority's legal department could be extremely significant. Nevertheless we were not aware of the existence of any guidelines within social services departments relating either to the appropriateness of a particular legal status in given situations or to the point at which the legal department should be consulted. The onus of identifying what advice might be valuable and whether an approach to the legal department might be appropriate was left to the social worker.

Choice of placement

Type of placement. In describing admissions based on the child's behaviour, we pointed out that in such admissions choice of type of placement was influenced by the assumption that adolescents were placed in residential care. In rescue from the family admissions, confidence in the value of foster care for young children was evident. Thus, of the 28 children aged under 11 years involved in these admissions, 21 were initially placed in foster care, whilst the six adolescents involved were placed in some form of residential care.

The high proportion of children placed in foster care reflects the distinct preference for this form of care expressed by the majority of workers. Asked why foster care had been selected, social workers indicated surprise that any other type of placement might be considered. For example, they said:

I wouldn't consider anything else for young children.

I think it's probably departmental policy to foster a child of this age.

This preference was also reflected in the period after admission in that those initially placed in residential care were moved to foster placements at the earliest opportunity. In these cases, admission had occurred at short notice and generally at hours inconvenient to foster parents, the child thus being placed temporarily in residential care.

The rationale for the selection of foster care was that it represented the closest approximation to 'normal family life' and as such was better than any other form of care. Foster placements were said to have been arranged 'in the interest of the child'. However, although we noted that the case for fostering in individual cases was made in these terms, we also noted when discussing the study child, social workers referred to children in general, rather than to the individual circumstances of specific children. For example, it was said:

> I would always go for foster care — normal family life is better than a children's home.

> I've always tried to avoid residential care. Foster care has so much more to offer even if the residential care is good.

Although little reference was made to the availability of resources in relation to type of placement, the choice of actual placement was influenced by assumptions about the scarcity of resources. As was pointed out in Chapter Two, the allocation of foster care resources in the study areas tended to be dealt with by a section at headquarters or a specially appointed officer in the area. Social workers seeking a foster placement were therefore unlikely to be directly or indirectly in control of resources. Although the study sample did not provide any instances of the request for a foster placement not being met, social workers did feel there was a likelihood of this occurring. Typical comments were:

> There is no choice — you have to take what you can get.

> There is such a shortage of foster homes, you don't quibble about what you are given.

Actual placement. Such was the strength of the assumption about the value of foster care that very few prerequisites were stipulated about the type of foster home required and indeed there was only one recorded instance of a first offer being refused as unsuitable.

It was not unusual, some time after placement, for social workers to volunteer praise about the placement. The positive features they identified included proximity to the parental home, the foster parents willingness to 'endure' parental contact and their ability to tolerate an open-ended duration for the placement. They appreciated, however, that these were characteristics coincidental to the decision to use the placement and not prerequisites of it.

In Care

It is apparent from the foregoing that the responsibility for arranging a child's placement in care rested largely with the worker dealing with the admission. Although the fact that someone else was more directly in control of resources meant that there were limitations on the choices available to the social worker, in practice the social worker's choice was generally met within the terms specified. The fact that placements appeared to be made on the basis of a generalised assumption about the value of foster care, as opposed to an assessment of individual placement needs, may, however be of more direct significance. In a later chapter, we examine the implications of making placements in this manner for the child's duration in care.

Parent-child contact. As with the case with child behaviour admissions, social workers rarely reported that decisions about parent-child contact had been taken at the time of admission. It was nonetheless apparent that in some cases decisions had been taken, albeit implicitly. For example whilst it was never stated at the point of admission that parental contact was to be discouraged, subsequently social workers did make the point that they had not actively encouraged it. Overall, their approach to parental contact was that of 'waiting to see what the parents do' and invariably the parents and foster parents were left to work out arrangements for contact between themselves. The initiative, in other words, was left with the parents, the social worker reacting and responding to the resultant situation.

We further noted that in securing placements, little consideration was given to the extent to which features of the placement might facilitate contact, or the contrary. Similarly there was little evidence of social workers providing parents with assistance to maintain contact.

The theme of decisions concerning parent-child contact arises at various stages of this report. Within the context of admissions of this type, we would draw attention to the fact that though social workers do not routinely address themselves to the issue at this point, is not to say that their approach had no effect. The fact that social workers 'leave it to the parents' is in itself taking a decision on parent-child contact.

Service to the family admissions (n=28)

Who takes the decision to admit?

Our data on what happens in service to the family admissions is rather more restricted since this type of admission was more likely to be dealt with by an intake or duty worker. By the time of our first interview, some of the cases involved had been transferred to a further social worker and the information obtained was therefore secondhand. However, as far as we were able to ascertain, these decisions are not dealt with in a substantially different manner from those based on the notion of rescue from the family.

Here, the influence and pressure of other agencies was not present but parents were often described as exerting a pressure of their own: they were said to have stated that they had 'no place to turn' and that 'they didn't know how they would manage if social services didn't take the children'. Several parents threatened to abandon the children in the department if no action was taken.

There were, however, no instances of admission being preceded by case conferences and indeed the discussions which did occur were described as informal and having involved either the team leader or another team member. Essentially the function of such discussions was 'keeping the team leader informed of what was going on' and not that of seeking authority to arrange admission. Thus, although our data are restricted to actual admissions, they do suggest that, when presented with a 'potential' admission, social workers tend first to establish whether they feel admission is appropriate; if so, they proceed with admission, possibly first approaching their team leader, recommending this action. Such recommendations, however, appear to be rarely refused and overall it seemed that the cases discussed were those which social workers judged should be admitted, those which social workers thought were inappropriate candidates for care not being referred for discussion.

The process involved in admissions of this type was therefore much less formal than that suggested by the various admission procedures and arguably the social worker was even more likely than in the other two types of admission to be the key decision maker.

Choice of legal status

Each of the 28 admissions based on the notion of service to the family was admitted to voluntary care. In general, no consideration was given to any other type of legal status since according to the social worker concerned 'there was no real concern for the future'. Three cases were exceptions to this. Whilst they were voluntary admissions, the children involved had been in care on several previous occasions and there was some anxiety about the care they were receiving at home. However, since the parent(s) were requesting care, voluntary care was organised in an effort to ensure that parental co-operation continued. Overall, there appeared to be general acceptance that voluntary care was the appropriate vehicle for admitting children in the circumstances of providing a service to the family.

Choice of placement

Six of the 28 admissions were placed on admission in residential care, four of these involving children aged over 11. In each of the six a preference was expressed for foster care but either because the child was part of a sibling group entering care and it was felt that the group should remain together, or because foster care would cause unnecessary disruption to schooling, placement in residential care occurred.

In terms of selecting both type and actual placement, our data revealed much the same findings as those in relation to rescue from the family admissions: foster care was valued more than residential care, on the assumption that in general it provided a better environment for children, and although subject to real and perceived resource constraints, the selection of placement was made by social workers. In one respect, however, service to the family admissions differed: child and parent(s) were generally introduced to the placement prior to the admission occurring. Although this did not amount to either parent or child participating in the selection of placement, it was a practice stressed by social workers when it occurred. The planned nature of these admissions meant that there was adequate time for this activity, highly valued in the professional literature, and as well as reducing the stress of later separation for the child, social workers felt that it reassured the parents: 'it helps the parents I think — even if they don't see them (the children), they can visualise where they are and feel confident that they are being cared for'. Undertaking this activity would also appear to underline the service to the family aspect of these admissions which set them apart from the other two main admission types.

Parent-child contact

Once again, as with other types of admission, it was the exception rather than the rule for social workers to report that any decision had been taken about parent-child contact. In general, when asked, social workers replied that it had been left to the parents and foster parents to work out a mutually acceptable arrangement and in any event the care duration was expected to be brief in these admissions. In a number of instances, there were, of course, additional barriers to contact in the sense that the admission occurred because a single parent was entering hospital. In one such case, however, the placement was selected on the understanding that the foster mother agreed to take the children to visit their mother in hospital. This case was exceptional and in general, social workers' involvement in decisions about parent-child contact was considerably more indirect.

Summary

In this chapter, each of the three main types of admission has been examined in terms of the decisions which must be taken as a child enters care, and the question 'who takes these decisions?' and on what basis has been asked. Despite the different underlying reasons for care and the responsibilities thus placed on local authorities in each type of admission, in the context of decision-making, admission types were fundamentally similar.

As far as the decision to admit is concerned, it is apparent that within social services departments a key role is undertaken by main grade social workers. Basically, it was they who determined who entered the department's care system, although it must be added that they rarely executed this task feeling that they had any alternative, and often only after long and sustained pressure from other agencies or even from the child's family. Likewise, the other decisions taken on admission, those concerning the child's legal status, placement and so forth, were left to be dealt with by the social worker, although once more other agencies and personnel might exert an influence and restrict the actual choices open to social workers. At the time of admission, then, main grade social workers have considerable scope to influence what happens to individual children.

The chapter has also highlighted that in taking decisions at admission, social workers are guided by generalised assumptions about the appropriateness of certain actions in relation to specific situations. Cases become 'categorised' according to criteria such as age, underlying reason for admission and the need for control, in such a way that decisions about legal status and placement were made in a 'routine' manner and not necessarily with reference to the child's individual set of circumstances. Whilst legal status and placement decisions could have significant implications for the child's future relations with his family, social workers rarely relayed that they had taken decisions at the point of admission about parent-child contact. However, whether described as a decision or not by social workers, leaving the initiative for contact with the parents was in itself a decision which undoubtedly had implications for the child in care.

CHAPTER FIVE
What Enables Discharge From Care?

The links between admission type and length of time in care were explored in Chapter Three. In this chapter, the circumstances in which individual children leave care are examined from the perspective of decision-making. Children may leave the care system by one of three routes: their care may be resumed by their birth parent(s); they may be adopted and acquire new parents; or they may remain in the care system until they reach the age of 18 (or exceptionally 19) at which age they are legally no longer children.

Of the 204 care episodes in the study period, there was a total of 81 discharges from care involving 71 children (8 children having at least two separate care episodes). Table 5:1 sets out the routes by which these 81 discharges occurred according to the type of admission.

Table 5.1
Exit route from care by admission type

Exit from care	Service to family	Child behaviour	Rescue from family	Other	Total
Care resumed by parents	29	21	17	2	**69**
Child attained 18-19	3	3	1	–	**7**
Adoption	–	0	3	2	**5**
Total care episodes ending	**32**	**24**	**21**	**4**	**81**
Total care episodes in sample	**54**	**66**	**74**	**10**	**204**

Care resumed by parents

Service to the family admissions (n=29)

A characteristic of family service admissions was the expectation as they entered care that normal family life would shortly be resumed. In fact, over 40 per cent (29) of all cases where care was resumed by parents in the study period were family service admissions, the vast majority (24 of the 29) leaving within two months of admission. With three exceptions, these discharges were achieved without active social work involvement, in the sense that the children concerned left care without the participation of their social workers, and often without their prior knowledge. The case of Hannah illustrates what typically occurred.

> Hannah's admission to care with a brother and sister was organised because of and in advance of her mother's admission to hospital for an operation. Two weeks after she entered care, we were informed of Hannah's return home by the social worker, who said 'I heard through the foster mother, who had taken the children to hospital to visit their mother, that mother was likely to come out in the next few days. The next thing I knew was the foster mother phoned to say that the mother had collected the children that evening at tea time'.

In the three 'exceptional' cases, the social workers were more actively involved: in one instance, by attempting to dissuade the mother from removing the child from care, and in two by exerting pressure on the parents to take their child back.

The remaining five family service admissions who returned home, had spent considerably longer in care and indeed their leaving care at that time was somewhat less expected. The circumstances of one of these discharges had much in common with the discharges described above, in that the boy returned to live with his father after two years in care without informing the social worker of his plans. In two cases, the social services department were directly involved in returning home children whom it appeared were being abandoned in care. In each case, changes in the children's in-care situation and the recent reallocation of the cases appeared to be significant factors in facilitating the children's return. For example:

> Deborah was admitted to care as a baby to enable her single parent

mother to complete her vocational training, Deborah being placed
with foster parents. Although her mother completed her training, she
did nothing to have Deborah back and indeed left the area. Several
years passed and throughout this period mother's contact with
Deborah was irregular and contact with the social worker was
maintained through the foster mother. Just prior to the study period,
it became known that mother was planning to return to her homeland
abroad and at approximately the same time, the foster mother
announced that she was not prepared to care for Deborah on a long-
term basis. The case had been unallocated for some time but at this
point was re-allocated. Working closely with her team leader, the
new social worker put it to mother that unless progress was made
towards Deborah's return, alternative plans would be made and her
access might have to be withdrawn. Mother confirmed that she
continued to want Deborah back and, despite the fact that several
hundred miles separated the two, a time-limited plan of introductory
visits back home and intensive work with Deborah was put into
operation. Within months, mother and daughter were re-united and
after more than three years in care, Deborah went to live in mother's
country.

Zoe, a six-year-old and her four-year-old brother Dale were
admitted to care at their mother's request: her cohabitation had just
broken up and she felt unable to cope with the children single-handed.
At the start of the study period, when the children had already been
in care for several months, the social worker described mother's
contact with the children as irregular and unsatisfactory but stated: 'If
mother asks for them, we'll have to let them go back. I am not saying
it would last but I think we'd have to give her a chance.'

Shortly thereafter, the foster mother demanded Zoe's removal but
said she was prepared to keep Dale. Accordingly, Zoe was moved to
another foster placement. The social worker then left the
department and the case was unallocated for some time. During this
period the team leader decided to review the case and invited mother
to the office to enquire of her plans. On hearing that she still wanted
to have the children returned but no longer had accommodation, he
wrote to the Housing Department supporting a priority nomination
and encouraged the mother to visit regularly to demonstrate her
seriousness about the children's return. He then allocated the case
and when mother was re-housed, the new social worker assisted her
in furnishing her home. After more than a year in care, the children
returned home.

Finally in two cases, the children's return to the parents was definitely not foreseen, and was in fact quite contrary to social work plans. Although both cases (one a single child, the other a sibling group of three), had originally been service to the family admissions, it had long been assumed within the social services departments concerned that the children would not be returning home and parental rights had therefore been assumed. Moreover, action had been taken to secure long-term foster placements with the possibility of adoption in the future. From the point of view, then, of the social services departments concerned, the cases had become rescue from the family type cases. Thus, when on the basis of different legal grounds, a parent in each case appealed to the courts, their action was opposed by the social services departments. In both instances the courts ruled in favour of the parents and the children returned home. Here, then, again, it was the action of the parents (albeit with the support of the court) which directly enabled discharge from care.

Child behaviour admissions (n = 21)

Thirty per cent of the cases whose care was resumed by parents were originally child behaviour admissions. All the children involved were over 11 years old when they entered care and 15 of the 21 had been admitted to voluntary care. However although care was technically assumed by the parents not all the young people involved actually returned to the family home; one joined the Armed Forces, two were held in penal establishments and transferred to the probation department, and three had made their own domestic arrangements.

Many of the 15 voluntary admissions involved girls, whose care episodes rarely exceeding six months. In general, the young person's discharge was preceded by some form of reconciliation between the young person, and his or her family. As with the majority of service to the family discharges, these young people tended to leave care without their social workers knowing until after the event. Dinah's case is typical:

> Dinah was admitted to care only after extreme pressure on the social worker by her parents: she was staying out all night, spending her time in 'bad' company, and missing school. After three weeks in care, she began to make occasional visits home and was accepted by parents. On one such visit, they suggested that she should just remain at home.

Dinah agreed and a telephone call was made to the residential unit where she was placed to arrange the collection of her belongings the following day. When this occurred, the residential staff informed the social worker who then recorded Dinah's official discharge from care.

The six cases who had entered care compulsorily presented a rather different picture. The final decision in these was, of course, that of the court discharging the care order but in all instances this had been recommended by the social worker involved. However, closer examination of the events preceding the child leaving care revealed that the social worker had not always initiated the process of discharge. In three cases, certainly, the social worker approached the court for the discharge of the care order: two of these being cases of young people held in penal establishments and where the local probation department had agreed that they would deal with the young person's after-care on licence, and the third being that of a girl who refused to have anything at all to do with the social services department. Since the social worker was leaving the department and the girl was already over 16 years old, the social worker applied to the court for the discharge of the care order. In the remaining three cases, the young person or parent approached the social worker seeking advice on how to have the care order removed, and in each case the social worker then supported this step in court, but they themselves had had no intention of taking action to discharge the order until such time as it was suggested by the client. In other words though social workers were involved in the process of the child leaving care they were not, strictly speaking, initiators of this.

Rescue from the family admissions (n = 17)

Approximately 25 per cent of the instances where care was resumed by a parent or parents had initially been rescue from the family admissions. Seven of these involved the straightforward process already described: the parent or parents removed the child or the child returned home with no involvement by the social worker, who often learned of the discharge only once it had occurred. Since these cases had been voluntarily admitted to care, the parents had retained the power to do this. A further four cases involved a slight modification of this process: in three the child had been removed from the care of one parent, and care was later assumed by the other. Social work involvement in such discharges varied. Although some social workers gave the 'new' parents a great deal

63

of support in the preparations required to permit assumption of the child's care (alternative accommodation was invariably necessary and in one case guardianship proceedings had to be instituted), in each case it was the parent who approached the social worker with the proposition that she or he might take the child, and not vice versa. In other words, again social workers were not the initiators of the plan to discharge from care.

In four of the remaining six cases, the situations of the individual children differed greatly. However in all four the period preceding discharge was characterised by placement difficulties. In three cases notification by foster parents that they were no longer willing to keep the child led social workers to reconsider returning the child home and in the fourth, the social worker's agreement to the parents' plan to return to their native country with the child, a severely mentally handicapped teenager, despite the fact that they had had virtually no contact with him in the previous two years, was preceded by unsuccessful attempts by the social worker to find him a suitable home.

It had been expected, if not planned, in each of these four cases that the children would not return home. In endorsing the children's return home, social workers acknowledged that there was no significant change in the home situation but were prepared to reappraise the possibility of return home only in the sense that it represented a less detrimental alternative for the child to that of remaining in care. As one of these social workers put it:

> If he'd stayed in care, we were confident that his educational needs could be catered for — but otherwise, he was going to have to keep moving — probably from one children's home to another — and I suppose that eventually might have affected his schooling. OK now we don't know what will happen with his education but it seems likely he'll have a relatively stable home base. It's the lesser of two evils really.

The discharge from care of the remaining two cases in this category represent marked contrasts to each other. In both, the child's leaving care was initiated by the social worker but in each for quite different reasons. In one, discharge was largely an administrative affair whilst in the other, it was part of an overall scheme to plan the child's future. In the former case, unsuccessful attempts to find a long-term foster family for a group of three children, coupled with mother's continued interest in the children and recent remarriage resulted in the children returning to mother and her new husband on a trial basis, just a year before the start of the research. In the initial social work interview the social worker stated: 'There are no plans to go back to court yet: it's going really well but it was so bad before we have to be really sure this time. The parents know that'. Less than six months later, when the social worker was reviewing her caseload prior to leaving the department, it was agreed to apply to the court for the discharge of the order. 'The parents', she said 'were quite overcome when we told them what we were intending to do.'

The second case was reallocated just as the research began, the child by then having been in care for three weeks. The new social worker explained that in taking over the case, she had been informed that there was a history of abandoning the child, a toddler, with anyone who was prepared to have him and that it was expected he would now be abandoned in care. The social worker felt this was a totally unsatisfactory situation: there was little documentation in the file and the child was in voluntary care so she saw no immediate prospect of being able to plan for his future. She therefore approached the mother and suggested returning the child on the condition that the mother agreed to a programme of support specified by the social worker. The mother agreed and the child was duly returned to her. However on the recurrence of mother's behaviour, the social worker felt able to make a case in support of compulsory care, and a care order was subsequently made.

In other words, with the exception of this latter case, circumstances preceding the discharge of these rescue from the family admissions suggest that as with service to the family and child behaviour admissions, the initiative for leaving care is rarely that of the social worker.

Other admissions

The care of two of the seven 'other' admissions was resumed by their parents during the study period. Both reflect circumstances leading to discharge from care already described: one teenage girl left care when her mother took her home after the girl had been abandoned by her stepfather, and in the other case the boy, again a teenager, returned to his parents after his foster parents said they were no longer prepared to look after him.

Summary

The process by which the care of a child is resumed by his or her parents is, of course, an interactive process. It requires a willingness on the part of the parent(s) to have the child back and where the child is subject to compulsory care, the approval of the court is required. In planning and making decisions for children, social services departments and social workers are therefore bound by these factors. However, on the basis of examining the circumstances in which children in each of the admission types left care, it becomes apparent that a child's departure from care is rarely the planned act of the social worker. This is not to say that social workers disapproved of the child's return home but highlights that social workers rarely act purposefully to achieve this end. The attitude and persistence of parents, the in-care situation and the involvement of team leaders seem in this respect to be more significant factors.

Child attaining the age of 18-19 years

Discharge from care of children on account of their age is inevitable at the point in time at which it occurs and is not, as such, the result of a social work decision. That such children remain in care to the conclusion of childhood may, however, be the planned, or unplanned outcome of social work decision-making.

Of the seven study cases leaving care on account of their age, three had been admitted because of their behaviour and had spent at least three years in care; whilst the remaining four, between them, had spent more than 55 years in care. The three child behaviour admissions, all adolescents at the time of their entry to care, had been expected to remain in care till the age of 16 years at least. A considerable part of the care period of each had been spent in penal establishments and indeed all three remained there at the time of their discharge from care. Latterly there had been little social services department involvement in these cases and the social workers concerned explained they had made no attempt to discharge the care order because: 'It was easier just to leave it. Anyway, it meant that we were here if we were wanted'. Each of these young people appeared to have lost contact with home. The remaining four cases had likewise lost contact with their own families. The child in one such case had entered care as a young adolescent, as a rescue from the family admission. For some time, parental contact was discouraged as it upset the child and later the youngster made it known she did not wish further contact with home. On this basis her remaining in care till 18 years was planned and she received extensive material support to facilitate her move to independent living. The remaining three cases had entered care as service to the family admissions at a very young age and were subsequently deemed to have been abandoned in care. Although each was admitted to voluntary care, the local authorities concerned had since assumed parental rights and duties. In each, the child's remaining in care was primarily a reflection of the fact that their parents had made no effort to resume their care. As a social worker concerned with one of these children put it:

> I wouldn't say it was planned that she wouldn't go back home — or that she remained in care for that matter. It's just what happened'.

Adoption

The five children who left care by adoption did so before the age of five years. Although they had spent different lengths of time in care prior to their adoption, each had been in care since birth, all were white, and admitted to care as single children and were *not*, therefore, what are commonly referred to as 'hard-to-place' children.

Two of these cases come under the category 'other admissions', since their parents had approached the social services department prior to the child's birth stating their wish that arrangements should be put in hand for the child's adoption. The children were, then, admitted to care at birth, placed briefly with short-term foster parents and subsequently with potential adopters. In both cases, the child was adopted within a year of admission to care.

The remaining cases were rescue from the family admissions, but like the two first mentioned they entered care at birth. In these cases the social workers' knowledge of injury to or inadequate care of other children in the family in the past meant that even before the children were born, there were plans to seek care orders on them. However, although securing care orders on the children was intended to ensure their removal from home, permanent alternative care in the form of adoption was envisaged for only one. While adoptive parents were found for this child, he was placed with short-term foster parents and the case was transferred to a senior case worker, who explained: 'It's an adoption case and I've experience of that, that's why it was reallocated and given   **67** to me'. Soon after being placed with the short-term foster parents, they indicated to the social worker that they would like to keep the child on a long-term basis by continuing to foster him. They were informed that the child was available for adoption only. Thus, when an adoptive home was found, the boy was moved and, after an initial delay to investigate a suspected hereditary handicap, he was subsequently adopted.

In the other two cases, the social workers in touch with the family prior to admission and responsible for admission, continued to be responsible for the children once they entered care. Again both were very experienced workers and said that at that time they envisaged the children remaining in long-term care. Suitable foster homes were therefore located prior to admission and the children moved, as infants, from hospital to long-term foster homes. In neither case was adoption part of the contract with foster parents, and indeed in both cases the social workers reported the placements were made without referring to this topic. According to them, the subject had never arisen, because whilst in general they thought that adoption would be ideal for the children, they felt it highly unlikely that the parents would ever grant their consent to such a step. Clearly then it was planned, or expected, that both children would remain in care long-term.

Examination of the events preceding the plan of adoption highlights once more the effect the child's in care situation can have on ultimate outcomes for children. In one of the cases, the foster parents, who had no family of their own, looked after the child for more than three years and then raised with the social worker the possibility of their adopting the child. In the second, the child was placed with foster parents who did have their own family and again had been with them for approximately three years when the child's birth mother wrote to the social worker saying she felt the child should be adopted. The social worker conveyed this to the foster parents on her next routine visit to them and although they immediately stated that they would like to adopt the child, the social worker stressed she had not been attempting to pressurise them towards adoption. She reassured them that, notwithstanding mother's letter, she planned that the child would remain with them and that although she would be delighted should they wish to adopt, the child would not be moved from them in order to achieve adoption.

In both cases the social worker concerned subsequently provided support and guidance to the foster parents which undoubtedly assisted them during the adoption process. However, theirs was a mediating role and the significant factor in processing the outcome of adoption for the child was the foster parents' decision to adopt and not social work planning.

Thus although only a few adoptions occurred in the study period, those that did suggested that the role of social work planning and decision-making was relatively insignificant. In contrast, factors such as the adoptability of the child — young, placed since infancy and not with siblings, the attitudes and circumstances of foster parents and the perceived and real attitudes of birth parents appeared to be highly significant, and to constitute situations to which social workers then responded.

Finally, one point is worth making in relation to all discharges from care. Although only a minority of discharges are effected by initiatives from within the social services department, the social worker carrying the case, as in other aspects of children's care careers, was the central social services department figure. Whilst the child's discharge from care might be discussed within a statutory review, the review itself did not take this decision. Likewise although 'discharge' meetings sometimes took place in Children's Homes, these occurred once it was clear the child was leaving care and were concerned with the after-care management of the case. However, having said that the case holder was the central figure, it is perhaps also noteworthy that in three cases, one leading to adoption and two to return home, the period of working towards the child's discharge was preceded by a re-allocation of the case. In transferring the case, the team leader outlined the plan for leaving care and worked closely with the social worker in achieving this. Given that the circumstances of the children involved in these cases were not dissimilar to many of those children who remained in care, this association would seem to be of some significance. There is some non-quantitative evidence to suggest that social workers valued this close working relationship on individual cases. Those considering the restructuring of service delivery might thus find this a fruitful avenue to explore.

Summary

In this chapter the circumstances in which individual children leave care has been examined in some detail. Regardless of admission type and the specific route by which children left care, there was little evidence to suggest that social workers purposefully worked towards children's exit from the care system. Indeed in many instances there was no social work involvement in the child's discharge, parents and children being the direct initiators of change. Where social work involvement was more in evidence, and although in individual cases it clearly did facilitate the child's return home or movement to a new permanent home, it was quite apparent that this involvement emerged in response to, or was prompted by, changes in the circumstances of the child's in-care situation. Case examples have highlighted the importance in this respect that foster parents' views of individual children may have on the eventual outcome for these children. Since at the time of entry to care social workers demonstrated a basically negative attitude to care, it is surprising, if not a matter of some concern, that the balance of factors contributing to children leaving care should be so heavily weighted towards factors other than social work involvement. The theme of how social workers plan their involvement in children's care careers is taken up in the next chapter.

CHAPTER SIX
Planning in Child Care

In Chapter One we pointed to the emphasis placed on the importance of planning, and particularly early planning, in the literature on child care. We likewise indicated that many regarded the inclusion of the welfare principle in the recent legislation concerning children in care as implying that an active and explicit approach to planning for children should be adopted. In general parlance, the terms 'planning' and 'decision-making' are often used interchangeably and in the context of child care few have defined what is meant by planning for children and how it may be distinguished from decision-making. One exception to this is Parker (1971) who defines planning for children as 'having a reasonably clear practical view of the future we wish for them and taking a sequence of steps which is instrumentally relevant to that end'. In this sense, planning may be viewed as 'anticipatory decision-making' occurring when the 'decision-maker is attempting to affect the future' (Drezner, 1973) and decisions may be seen as more specific events normally taken within the context of an overall plan. The activity of planning, therefore, encompasses notions of defining aims and objectives and then developing strategies to achieve these.

Intellectually, the potential association between the length of time a child spends in care and planning is self-evident and it was to this end that a considerable amount of research time was spent both in asking social workers about their plans and the foundation for them and in observing how plans were developed and the influence of stated plans. The purpose of this chapter is not simply to recount how social workers described their plans but to examine the nature of planning in practice and to consider the implications of this for children in care.

Planning as an activity at admission

The 114 new admissions to care during the study period enabled us to consider the extent to which planning takes place in the early stages of a child's career in care. We assumed that plans would probably be tentative in these early stages but thought that since our initial interview generally took place a few weeks after admission that by that time, social workers would have begun to formulate general views about the prospects of the child's return home or otherwise as a basis for their current work with the case.

In almost ten per cent of the admissions, the child had already left care by the time of this interview. In approximately three quarters of the remainder there were no clear plans. In these instances replies to the question 'What are your plans for this case?' fell into three categories, representing to some degree a continuum in the development of plans.

In the first of these, replies to questions about plans characteristically began: 'I would hope . . .', or 'I would like to think . . .'. Such replies were most commonly applied to the service to the family type of admission and reference was made to the likelihood of the child returning home. Although these statements were made in relation to specific children, the rationale for 'the plan' was given in terms of statements of the general principle of keeping families together. For example it was said:

> Well that's his home — I've got to try and make sure he goes back there.

> We always like to think that children will go back home.

Moreover, although a preferred course of action was outlined, most commonly the child's return home, there was little evidence of social work action in support of this, or recognition that in the absence of supporting action, the reverse might occur. For example, there were few instances of parents being actively assisted in the problems which resulted in the child's admission to care, it being said 'the parents will deal with that'. In addition, as was mentioned in Chapter Four, few positive measures were taken by social workers to ensure or facilitate contact between children and parents.

A second type of reply began: 'I imagine . . .' or 'I think it most likely . . .' and continued by outlining an expected outcome. This reply was characteristic of many child behaviour admissions, particularly those entering care on care orders, the outcome being expressed in terms of the length of time the child was likely to remain in care. For example, it was said:

> He is on a care order now so that's really him until he's completed his education.

I'm not sure whether he'll be in care until 18. A couple of years probably — when he is through full-time school.

The plans for 23 of the 28 child behaviour admissions admitted on care orders were expressed in this manner, indicating an assumption that the young person would remain in care until school leaving age at least. Such replies were given, then, in terms of the social workers' assessment of what was *likely* to happen, as opposed to what they felt *should* happen.

A third type of reply indicated that the social worker had not yet reached the stage of those above: they had not 'read' the situation sufficiently to allow them to 'predict' the likely outcome. Typically replies began:

We'll have to wait and see . . .
I'll have to see how things go . . .
It depends what the parents do . . . and It's too early to say — you can't tell at this stage.

Plans in relation to more than half the rescue from the family admissions were expressed in this manner.

Although social workers' tentativeness at this early stage is understandable, it meant that these workers had no overall view to guide them and the lack of this had repercussions for all concerned in the child care network, children, parents and social workers. For example, cases characterised by the absence of plans were also characterised by a limited, if not negligible, input of work with children and families. In other words, although a preferred or expected outcome was outlined, there was scant evidence of consistent social work action in support of this or recognition that such action might be necessary (see also Rowe and Lambert, 1973; Thorpe, 1974; Aldgate, 1976; Thoburn, 1980; and Hoelgaard, 1984). In discussing similar findings, Hoelgaard (1984) has described the differential provision of services to families as 'arbitrary'. The repercussions of this arbitrariness in individual cases is made apparent by the following case histories, where although the circumstances of the families were broadly similar, the approach of the social workers differed.

Case one: Planned returned home

In this case a six-year-old girl and her four-year-old brother were admitted to care from their pregnant mother and her cohabitee to allow the parents the opportunity of finding new accommodation. **73**

The mother had previously been evicted from her local authority home and had moved in with relatives but the strain of joint living was causing many problems.

At the time of the children's admission, the social worker stated: 'The plan is that they'll go back home — that's what the parents want and, I've no reason to think otherwise'. The mother accompanied the children to the children's home, was introduced to the staff and arranged to visit the children every third day after school.

For two weeks, the social worker did not contact the parents but made a weekly call at the children's home from whom she heard news of the children and of the parents' visits. In the third week, she visited the mother in her accommodation and heard that although she and her cohabitee had found a number of suitable places they had been unable to accept them because of the cost.

Because of the strain in relationships in the current home, the mother spoke of taking on a room elsewhere and leaving the children in care meantime.

The social worker said she hoped this wouldn't be necessary. The following day she contacted the housing department and was informed of the possibility of temporary accommodation becoming available. She informed the mother of this and, although at first reluctant, the mother eventually agreed to consider this option. Three days later, she telephoned the social worker saying she'd been offered a place but was not happy with it. The social worker arranged to meet the mother at the flat the following day. The social worker agreed that the flat was less than ideal but pointed out that she might be able to help with second-hand furniture and the family could be together again. Mother and her cohabitee agreed to think it over. The social worker heard nothing.

After a week had passed, she visited the mother at the relatives' home and discovered that they had turned the offer down and had found nothing else themselves. Their financial situation was then discussed and the social worker pointed out that any private accommodation the parents could afford was unlikely to be any better than that provided by the local authority. The parents agreed to go back to the housing department. After refusing a further offer they accepted accommodation and the social worker helped them to obtain second-hand furniture. The children were discharged home within seven weeks of admission.

Case two: 'Hoped' that the child would return home

Two sisters were admitted to care at their mother's request to allow her to sort herself out. A single parent, she had been helped by the social worker in the past with budgeting advice but now found herself about to be evicted and with many substantial debts.

When asked about her plan, the social worker said: 'I'm hoping they'll go back'. These children were placed in a foster home and it was arranged that the mother could visit on Saturdays to take the children out. The social worker did not contact the mother but telephoned the foster mother after a few days. The children were said to have settled down very well. In subsequent telephone calls or visits to the foster home, the social worker learned that the mother visited regularly and the children were settled.

At the end of the study year when the children were still in care, the social worker said 'I don't really have any plans. Mother sees the children regularly but she says she's not ready to have them back. She was young when she had them and I think she is enjoying the freedom now. I think what she is thinking is that she'll have them back when they are a bit older'.

Case three: Expected that the children would return home

A mother of two children, aged six and four, approached the department seeking care for the children whilst she 'sorted herself out'. She had considerable arrears of rent and debts with the fuel boards and her emotional life was in a state of some turmoil. The department agreed to the children's admission and placed them separately in two foster homes. The social worker stated she expected the children to return to their mother as she had indicated that care would only be temporary.

In giving mother the addresses of the foster homes, the social worker informed her that she should make arrangements to visit directly with the foster parents, a move which the social worker felt was a positive indication of her conviction that the children should return home.

There was then no contact between mother and social worker. Mother attempted to resolve some of her problems by relinquishing the tenancy on her council home and went to live with a friend. Her contact with the children became irregular and infrequent. Increasingly one of the foster mothers complained of the daughter's behaviour.

In a research interview about four months after admission the social worker said: 'I'm not sure what is going to happen — it looks like we have a long-term case on our hands — mother is not visiting and although I've not seen her myself, I know she's given up her house and presumably she has no home to offer them. It doesn't look good'.

Case four: 'Don't know — wait and see'

After being evicted from the family home, a mother of two children, recently separated from her husband, asked for her children to be admitted to care. Bed and breakfast accommodation was offered instead and mother accepted. After a few weeks she said she could tolerate that no more and it was eventually agreed the children would be admitted to care. They were placed in a foster home.

Asked at this time about her plans, the social worker replied: 'I don't know what will happen, it could go either way. I'll have to wait and see'. Although she had no contact with mother, she visited the children in foster care and confirmed that there were no difficulties.

When the children had been in care for almost six weeks, mother came to the department and informed the social worker of her address, adding that she hoped to have the children back soon and that she had been visiting them approximately every ten days. There was then no more contact for several weeks when the foster mother relayed to the social worker that when mother had last visited she had brought a friend and told the children that he would be living with them when they returned home.

At the second research interview the social worker said: 'I'm not sure what's going to happen — I haven't seen mother but I understand there were three weeks between her last visit to the children'. By this time, the children had been in care for more than five months.

Cases two, three and four just described lend weight to the findings of several studies carried out in the United States (see, for example, Gottesfeld, 1970) which have demonstrated that children become 'lost'in the child care system because parents became 'lost'. According to such writers, the syndrome of children drifting in care without firm plans is directly attributable to the failure to work with parents from the outset of the care episode.

Here the relative absence of social work input to parents in the early stages of children's care careers was rather surprising since even those social workers who had no plans made it clear that they viewed the parents as crucial in determining what happened to children. For example, in 55 of the 62 rescue from and service to the family admissions, social workers phrased their replies to questions about plans in the first research interview in terms of the parents. Broadly speaking, the implication was that in service to the family admissions, it was the wishes of the parents which would determine whether the child remained in or left care, whilst in rescue from the family admissions it was the parents' behaviour. In child behaviour admissions, especially those involving older children, slightly more emphasis was placed on the wishes and behaviour of the child, assuming, of course, the parents' willingness to have the child back.

The paradox that social workers could simultaneously stress the importance of parents and yet not actively work with them may appear confusing. For the social workers concerned, having no plans or 'waiting to see' implied that they were bringing no influence to bear and that they were somehow neutral actors in the situation. Clearly this is a misconception: by doing nothing one may still influence a situation. Social workers, who believed that by not actively encouraging an outcome, they were bringing no influence to bear, deceived themselves and were likely, albeit inadvertently, to be being passively discouraging.

However because there were no clear plans in the early stages of the vast majority of admissions is not to suggest that planning from the outset is impracticable. Indeed the few instances of positive planning encountered in the sample cases tended to be found in the early stages of childrens' care careers. Thus although the cases outlined below were exceptional, they graphically depict the substantial difference in approach of those with and without an overall view to guide them.

Martin's case

Social services were alerted to the case of three-week-old Martin when his parents' neighbours reported to the GP that they had twice found Martin's mother attempting to suffocate him. Martin had been placed in their care during the day by his father because his depressed mother would not attend to him. Martin was immediately removed to a local authority foster home and a few days later his mother was admitted to hospital with post-natal depression.

Working in close consultation with the hospital staff and the foster mother, the social worker arranged for Martin to be taken to hospital each day to spend some time with his mother. At the time of the first research interview, by which time his mother had been discharged home, the social worker described her plans in the following way:

'From the start I've been working towards his going back home eventually. His father is actually fairly pessimistic about it and has talked about adoption but I think it was quite a shock to him to see how his wife behaved. I've encouraged him to keep in contact with them both and mother has been allowed increasingly long periods of supervised contact with Martin. She's really only now starting to show any great interest and motivation and I am encouraging that as much as possible, whilst still protecting Martin, in the sense that there is always somebody else there. Mum is now home so she can go to the foster home during the day and I've informed foster mother that she can gradually start to leave the room a bit to see how mum gets on on her own. If that's OK we'll let her take him out for a few hours — that sort of thing. It's slow but it's going OK.'

By the time Martin was four months old, he had been discharged from care and returned home to live with both his parents.

Neil and Pauline's case

The social services department took a place of safety order on Neil aged six and Pauline aged four after they had been abandoned by their mother with neighbours for the fifth time in two years. Court proceedings were subsequently initiated and care orders obtained on both children. They had been in care four months when the social worker concerned gave the following account of his plans:

'The plan was dependent on the care order really. As you know these kids have been in and out of care and mother had been quite firmly told that if this happened again, we'd have to make alternative arrangements for them which wouldn't include her. When I heard about this last episode, I therefore placed the children in a children's home — so that they didn't form too many close ties — and started the search for prospective adoptors. Of course, I couldn't do very much till we got the care order, but when I traced mother I told her all this.

She says she wants them back even although we've been to court now and I've explained we are definitely opposed to that. I've allowed her to visit every week but I am now going to change that — I warned her I would — because I've now found a possible couple to adopt and introductions will begin next week. I am quite convinced these children's interests are not being served at home and I am doing what I can to provide an alternative'.

By the end of the research period, the children were placed with this couple who were in the process of applying to adopt. Since mother was against adoption and still saying she wished to have the children back, social services were preparing a case to dispense with her consent.

In both these cases the social worker's approach was not simply characterised by a vague notion of what might happen in the future but by a clear view of what *should* happen and by definite strategies designed to expedite the overall objective. By contrast, most social workers adopted a pretermitting approach to planning: that is they 'put off' engaging in planning and in so doing they failed to address the question of children's futures.

Planning as an activity at subsequent stages of children's care careers

The subsequent care careers of these new admissions as well as the care careers of the children who had already been in care for some time at the start of the research (the in-care sample) provided little evidence to suggest that planning becomes a much more prominent activity as time progresses. Indeed in a few cases (less than ten per cent) social workers insisted that there were no plans. In two instances the social workers claimed that given the circumstances of the cases (both involving adolescents) planning was inappropriate and although they described their approach as positive non-intervention, they did not appear to view this as synonymous with planning. In the remainder, it was claimed that it was generally unprofessional to plan because in child care one had to be responsive to changing circumstances. As one social worker put it 'There are no plans here. There never have been. You have to be open-minded in these matters. I'm a firm believer in being flexible.'

However most social workers did subscribe to the notion of planning, a 'plan' being outlined in 192 cases (90 per cent) of those under consideration. Nonetheless close examination of the plans stated suggested that exceptional though it was to express the viewpoint that one should deliberately not plan, this was in fact how many social workers behaved. In other words, although social workers used the vocabulary of planning, the plans they stated were not necessarily the outcome of a conscious planning process.

Indeed it was apparent that aspects of the social work approach identified at the time of the child's admission to care continued to feature even when the child had been in care some time. For example, in many instances stated plans still contained a predictive element, with replies to question about plans being prefaced 'what seems likely . . .', 'I am assuming . . .' and 'it looks like . . .'. Furthermore, social workers' explanations of their current plans suggested that they continued to see their function *vis-a-vis* parents as that of giving them scope to demonstrate their intentions and capabilities. The following quotations illustrate how in the absence of initiatives from parents, social workers tend to see the only option for children as that of being in care:

> Of a five-year-old in care since she was two with two siblings, it was said:
> I don't see there is any alternative (to care). The parents have done nothing to have them back. They visit but that is about it and if anything their own situation is worse now than when the kids came into care.

> And of a seven-year-old boy in care with his sister since he was five and a half:
> In the past she (the mother) has seemed quite happy to have the kids drift in and out of care. It's been much longer this time and she has shown no sign of having them back at all — that's why I am now looking for long-term foster homes for them.

> Of a ten-year-old in care since she was a year old:
> What's the alternative? There was a contact arranged with mother when she was about five. That was done by the social worker who held the case at that time and since then, there has been no contact that I am aware of. I don't even know where the mother is.

> Of a 15-year-old in care since five:
> I think for a long time we weren't sure what father was going to do — we never dealt with mother. Now it is quite clear father isn't interested — he's made his life and regrettably, Mark has to be in care.

These cases also highlight a feature evident in the case histories of many children in care for significant proportions of their childhood: that it may take a long time before a clear view emerges of the prospects of the child's return home. Such case histories typically contained statements about the unlikelihood of return home but rarely statements that the child would not be returning home. The plans stated in relation to children during this interregnum tended therefore to be reflections of the current situation, rather than plans as such.

However the most generally conspicuous feature of stated plans at subsequent stages of children's care careers was the extent to which the child's in-care situation predominated. This was evident in several respects and appeared to reflect a social work pre-occupation with 'in-care-ness'. For example interviews were carried out with social workers on 143 cases where the child had been in care for at least three months. In more than 85 per cent of these, the social worker replied to questions about plans in terms of the child's placement in care, the following social worker responses to the question 'So what are your plans now for the case?' being typical:

> *Social worker:* 'I imagine he'll stay where he is for the present'
> *Interviewer:* 'Where is that?'
> *Social worker:* 'In the foster home.'

> *Social worker:* 'We don't plan to move her in the forseeable future.'

> *Social worker:* 'We'll have to think of moving him soon — the foster home is only approved for short term placements and he's been there for nearly four months.'

This pre-occupation with 'in-care-ness' was also evident in the fact that social workers tended to view the options for children as being solely those of 'home' or 'care'. In other words, despite the emergence nationally in the late seventies of a pro-adoption lobby, references to adoption as a potential outcome for children were rarely encountered in the sample cases and where they were, it was generally in the context of explaining why adoption was inappropriate in the particular circumstances. However, it was clear in several cases that adoption was, or in the past would have been an obvious option. Certainly, too, in at least four cases, the parents had obviated the need for the social workers 'to wait and see' what they did. These parents had come forward either recommending that their child be adopted or clearly stating that they did not wish the child's return. At the time each child was in a foster home and despite the fact that they were technically available for adoption, this option had not been raised with the foster parents or otherwise explored. At the study start, each of these children had been in care for at least three years but none was more than eight years old. Each was expected to remain in care throughout the remainder of their childhood.

In Care

Furthermore, it was evident that the single most significant factor in crystallising the social worker's view of the home situation was the perceived stability of the child's in-care placement, this being particularly marked where the child was in foster care. In other words, whilst in the period immediately following admission, the child's being in care was explained in terms of the parents, subsequent explanations increasingly focused on accounts of how settled the child had become in his/her foster home. The following brief case histories illustrate this point:

Bryan

The research involvement began with Bryan's admission to care aged ten months old. He'd been in care approximately four and a half months at the time of the second interview with the social worker.

When asked why the baby remained in care, the social worker said: 'He's settled so terribly well — they all love him there. It's difficult to remember him at home'.

In reply to the same question four months later, the social worker said: 'The parents would have to do something pretty spectacular now — to have him back. He's so settled there.'

And at the final interview, by which time there had been a change of social worker, the new social worker said: 'Why is he still in care? Well as I understand it, the parents have shown little indication that they plan to have him back and really he is so settled there, it would be criminal to move him.'

Bernard

Five-year-old Bernard had been in care for more than four years at the time the research began, At this stage, the reason for his remaining in care was given as 'He's been there (the foster home) for what . . . four years now, that's his home. You couldn't move him.'

And a year later, at the end of the research period, it was said, 'He's been there five years. That's his home — its not being in care to him. I suppose since there has been no contact with father, you could argue that he should be adopted but you just couldn't move him, that's his home and that's where he'll stay.'

Indeed such was the significance ascribed by social workers to children settling in foster care that within a relatively brief period it could counterbalance the earlier emphasis on parents and lead the social worker at least to question the original 'plan' that the child would return home. For example in one such service to the family admission, the social worker said in the initial research interview that she expected the child would probably be in care for about six months. The parent, a single mother had regular weekend contact with the child, who was in a foster home for the first eight weeks of the admission. Thereafter her contact became less frequent and irregular. When the child had been in care four months, the mother told the foster mother she had new accommodation and that she would be resuming care of the child herself within six weeks. Relaying this to us in the second research interview the social worker said:

> I'm really not quite sure what to do. The (foster parents) really love the kid and Matthew has thrived since he went there. You wouldn't believe he'd ever been anywhere else. It's voluntary care though and I don't know that I've got the power to stop her (the mother) having him.

According to several social workers, the fact that children 'settled' in foster care validated their earlier approach of 'waiting to see what happened with the parents'. We noted, however, that where the child was in any other form of care, or where the continuance of the foster placement was in any way in doubt, ambivalence about the child's prospects of return home could continue indefinitely. Furthermore, during the study period there were no less than nine separate instances of children having to be moved from what their social workers had described as long-term foster placements. In each of these, the child had been placed with the foster parents at a very early age and remained there for at least two years, and in some cases considerably longer. They left the placement because the foster parents demanded their removal.

To sum up so far, then, although with the passage of time social workers state plans for the children in their care, in practice these are rarely, regardless of admission type, the outcome of a conscious planning process. Indeed, in the majority of cases, the activity of planning appears to be continually postponed with social workers adopting a stance which can best be described as passive. However the passive stance of social workers, itself, sets in train a process of dealing with children which, in contrast to the planning process, is fundamentally reactive in nature. In this process, the 'plans' stated by social workers are first reflections of their reliance on parents to determine the outcome for children, and then, in the absence of initiatives from parents, of their propensity to view children's futures as being inevitably within the care system.

Influences on children's care careers

One of the consequences of dealing with children's care careers in the above manner is that there is increased scope for other influences on what happens to children. In this respect, we found that the child's caretaker in care and the courts could have a significant, though generally unrecognised and under-estimated impact.

Foster parents

Foster parents' attitude to keeping a child beyond a short-term period could be crucial to what subsequently happened to that child: their attitudes could determine whether the child went home, remained in care or was adopted.

It was evident, for example, that substantial numbers of children were allowed to continue indefinitely in the short-term placements in which they were placed on admission to care. Although we are unable to produce precise figures on this, some idea of the scale of this pattern may be conveyed by pointing out that such was the experience of at least 28 of the 185 sample children. Such cases were typified by social workers having reservations about the prospects of the child's return home, but doing little to confirm the situation either way unless, or until, such time as the foster parents indicated their willingness to keep the child. The following extracts from interviews with social workers illustrate how this occurs:

> As you (interviewer) know, I wasn't very sure what was really happening on the home front. I was feeling increasingly uneasy about it. I mentioned this in passing to the foster mother one day and she said they would love to keep him . . . so I suppose you could say that the plan is long-term care with these foster parents.

> What happened was that the foster parents said they would like to keep him — you know, long term — so we've gone along with that. I am quite happy with that because I didn't really see that (the parents) were ever going to have him back.

> The foster parents got in touch to say that James had been with them for more than six months and they didn't like to keep children that

long. Eventually I got hold of the parents and we agreed that if they could give an undertaking about hospital check-ups, we would allow James back home.

Furthermore in cases which had undergone this process and the plan for the child had come to be stated as 'long term care with these foster parents' social workers invariably continued:

We haven't raised it but what we are hoping is that in time the foster parents will want to adopt. Even if they don't, we'll not be moving him — he is so settled there.

This is not to say that such placements were originally made in the expectation or hope that adoption would follow. More commonly, the question of adoption arose considerably later, and generally at the initiative of the foster parents. Although in the following examples, some highly individual situations are involved, the approach of the social workers of acting only in response to initiatives by foster parents is typical:

Diane

At the time Diane, a young infant, was admitted to care, there was an acute shortage of short-term foster placements. However, despite the fact that the social worker had reservations about the particular foster parents offered for the child, she accepted the placement, it being the only one on offer. Other than accompanying the social worker to place Diane, mother did not visit and disappeared without notifying the social services department.

Although unhappy with the placement, the social worker did not attempt to find an alternative. When Diane had been with the foster parents for more than six months, they volunteered that they were prepared to keep Diane long-term. Later still, they stated they would like to adopt her. At the end of the study year, the social worker reported that no firm decision had been taken on either of these offers, but that Diane remained in the placement and that she had no plans to move her.

Christopher

At three years old, it appeared that Christopher had been abandoned by his single-parent mother at the nursery he attended. The social services department discovered within a month of his admission that **85**

In Care

Christopher's mother had died. On learning this, the short-term foster parents volunteered to keep Christopher on a long-term basis. From the time of the second research interview, the social worker talked of his optimism that the foster parents would eventually adopt. The subject of adoption was, however, never raised with the foster parents, despite the fact that they attended a number of reviews during the study period. At the end of the year, the social worker stated the plan for Christopher as remaining with the foster parents with hopes of adoption in the future. And the reasons for remaining in care as 'he is too settled to move'.

Darren

At six months old Darren was admitted to care on a care order, but in the early stages of the study he was returned to his mother on a trial basis. After a few months, she asked for him to be removed and since no other placement was said to be available, he was placed with a couple who had previously fostered his mother and who had continued to maintain an interest in her. It was Darren's mother who eventually suggested to the social worker that adoption would be best for Darren. According to the social worker, when she relayed this information to the foster parents, 'they seized on it'. By the end of the study their application to adopt the child had been lodged with the court.

In other words, as these examples show, what may determine whether a child remains in care with a foster family, or is adopted, can be the viewpoint of the foster parents and the extent to which they make their views known to the social worker. Given this context, 'the plans' subsequently stated had been formed in a reactive manner.

However it was clear that where foster parents were less favourably inclined towards keeping a child long-term, they did not always feel able to express this so readily. This was rarely picked up by the social workers and the child's placement in the foster family typically drifted from short to long term in an unplanned and certainly unagreed fashion. In the course of the study period, some foster parents with this experience were described as suddenly demanding the child's removal. In these circumstances it was not unusual to find the social worker then giving consideration to the possibility of the child returning home, even although there was very little parent-child contact and it had previously been suggested that return home was unlikely. The following were two

such cases.

Adrian

Adrian was admitted to care when he was two years old after being subjected on several occasions to non-accidental injury at the hands of his step-father. He was placed in a short-term foster home. Four years later, at the start of the research, Adrian was still with the same foster family, and in the previous year had had two contacts with his mother, both lasting only a few hours.

Asked about plans for Adrian, the social worker replied: ' He will stay where he is long-term. He is very much part of that family'. At the same time, however, we noted that over the years, the social worker had recorded in the file that from time to time the foster mother had commented on Adrian's slower than average development and rather unusual behaviour patterns.

During the study period the foster parents made it quite clear that they wished Adrian to be removed from the family as soon as possible. By the time of the final research interview Adrian had been placed 'temporarily' in a children's home to assess what should happen in the future. In that interview the social worker said 'what I am thinking at the minute is that perhaps we should try home now . . . I don't like the idea of residential care for what would be ten years. On the other hand, he is older now and he may not be at the same risk at home.'

Kevin

At six months old, Kevin was admitted to care and placed with short-term foster parents. At the start of the research, some three years later, the social worker stated that the foster parents appeared willing to keep Kevin long-term and 'I'm hoping that they will eventually want to adopt him.' Nonetheless towards the end of the research period, the foster parents said that they were not prepared for the placement to continue much longer and asked 'when can you find him somewhere else?'. The child was still with the foster parents at the end of the research period and the social worker stated 'I am not really sure what's going to happen. I have seen mother and I did raise Kevin with her — that may be a possibility now — I've arranged that he can spend a day with her at Easter.'

Both these cases involved single children in care but if anything the situation was even more marked if the child was part of a sibling group in care. Here the foster parents' wish to be relieved of a group or part of a family group could trigger off reassessments of both the home and in-care circumstances to such an extent that what was at one time

considered a totally unsatisfactory home situation came to be seen to be
'good enough' in view of the deterioration in the in-care situation. The
Williams case was one such instance:

The Williams children

The three Williams children were admitted to care during the study
period. From the start, the social worker expressed doubt that they
would ever return home. At the third research interview, she
reported that the parents had had very little contact with the children
and had shown very little interest in their future, she therefore felt
her earlier reservations were justified. In the final interview she
reported that she was very unhappy about the children returning
home but added that all three had deteriorated since being admitted
to care and that the two sets of foster parents were beginning to
enquire when the children would be removed. In the past month,
mother had also reappeared on the scene and although the home
situation had changed very little, the social worker said that the plan
was now that the children would return home. Explaining the reasons
for this change, the social worker said: 'sometimes you have to stop
and look and ask yourself — what are we doing to these children here?
We really haven't offered them much. I really feel they will be no
worse at home and mother seems quite keen to have them'.

The influence of foster parents, then, was such that it could result in a
range of outcomes for individual children. In the context of children's
futures what is perhaps more generally significant is the scale of the
influence which foster parents are able to bring to bear, albeit quite
inadvertently. That it is possible for them to do this is a function of the
reactive manner in which cases are handled.

Residential staff

The influence of caretakers from the residential sector was rather
different and tended to lead to changes in the in-care situation rather
than changes of overall status. For example, as far as young children
were concerned, residential staff could be powerful motivators in
securing foster families. Thus, in four study cases the search for foster
homes for sibling groups, in care at least a year, was initiated by
residential staff. Although the social workers in these cases were not
against the children moving to foster care, and indeed strongly disliked

the prospect of the children remaining in residential care, they had done little to pursue this course of action until pressured by the residential staff.

The influence of residential staff in relation to older children was in the direction of the children's return home, though not necessarily their discharge from care. Moreover, this outcome could be achieved despite social workers' reservations about home and return to the community. For example, a number of boys placed in community schools returned home at the age of 16 years as the school said they were discharging them. In most of these cases the social workers felt the boys were not ready for a return to the community and should be placed in some form of supervised placement. Nonetheless with termination of the community school placement they did not always seek an alternative.

Although a plan of return home was stated this evolved in response to the anticipated actions of the residential sector, rather than as a positively planned outcome. Likewise some adolescents returned home because the residential staff refused to tolerate their behaviour any longer and demanded the child's removal. In such cases the social worker would generally postpone the placement ending, stating that a further placement would first have to be found. Nonetheless, in reality discharge invariably followed. The following is a typical example:

Joe, a 14-year-old, had been in the same children's home for five years. The parents did not visit him but he occasionally went home for a few hours at the weekend. In a fit of temper, he assaulted a new member of staff and the staff of the home contacted the social worker demanding his removal. In discussing the matter with the social worker, Joe made it clear he wanted to remain in the home and not return to his parents. The social worker explained that it was impossible for Joe to remain where he was and that he, the social worker, would try to find something similar for him. He suggested that in the meantime, Joe might consider going home on a temporary basis. Joe reluctantly agreed.

A month later in a research interview, the social worker said: 'I should have been trying to find something for him but I must admit I haven't got round to it. He came in to see me yesterday and I said there was nothing, However, things seem to be going not too badly at home — at least he is still there, which is something — and I think I may just let things lie for a bit.'

At the next interview, the social worker told us that Joe was no longer living at home and that he, the social worker had not seen him for more than six weeks. He 'understood' that Joe was moving from squat to squat, occasionally living with friends' parents.

The Courts

The influence of the courts was less direct than that of foster parents and residential staff and had its origins in social workers' perceptions of what the courts generally expected rather than in explicit statements about individual children. In other words, stated plans were formed on the basis of what would be acceptable to the court.

This was particularly marked in relation to children on care orders, many of whom spent lengthy periods of care placed at home on a trial basis. Social workers' aforementioned propensity to assume that a child entering care as an adolescent was likely to remain in care until school leaving age was at least in some measure attributable to their perception that this was what the courts expected. Furthermore, social workers appeared to believe (perhaps justifiably) that the courts required certain minimum standards of behaviour in children and families before they would entertain the idea of discharging a care order. Thus although social workers might themselves be generally satisfied that a care order was no longer required, they had reservations that the court would agree: in consequence plans would be described as 'remaining in care meantime'. It was said, for example, of one 15-year-old who had been placed home on trial for over a year:

> I am quite happy with the arrangements at home and so I don't see Billy or his parents at all. But I can't get rid of the care order because his attendance is poor and the court would be horrified.

However the court's influence was not confined to child-behaviour-type admissions exclusively. This influence extended also to cases which had originally been rescue from the family admissions, and particularly those where sibling groups of children were involved. Explaining why one family group, living at home for the past four years, was likely to remain technically in care for the foreseeable future, the social worker said:

> There are a lot of problems there, there always will be but if there is one thing we've achieved it's mother's trust. She'll come to see us now if she has any worries — that makes an irrelevance of the care order and it would really make her day, if we took it back to court but they would never wear it . . . the background isn't too impressive.

In other words, although the court's influence was unlikely to be child-specific, its effect was to set potential outcomes within pre-defined parameters.

Thus, one of the consequences of deferring planning is that children's care careers tend to be moulded by the behaviour and attitudes of a number of adults who do not necessarily have any overall responsibility for the child. In this respect it is likely that the length of time a child spends in care is determined by factors which are, in a sense, quite 'happenstance' (Simon, 1957).

What inhibits planning?

It seems unlikely that the all too frequent lack of purposeful planning exemplified by the study cases can be cursorily dismissed as unprofessional conduct on the part of social workers simply because social workers have professionally been exhorted to engage in planning. However the potentially harmful and deleterious consequences for children of what in practice is referred to as 'planning' render it important to understand why social workers behave in the manner in which they do. In this respect, the data suggest that it may be necessary to look first at what happens even before a child is admitted to care.

The stressful nature of working with children and families

Entailing as it does highly complex family situations where the parents' motives and abilities are in question and where judgements have to be made about 'risk' to children, child care work is undoubtedly a highly stressful occupation. Furthermore all indications are that in the period immediately preceding admission to care, this stress is exacerbated: in many instances other agencies are pressurising for 'something to be done' and as has already been shown, the individual who has to deal with this, as well as with the complicated mechanics of admission, is the social worker. The stress experienced by social workers at this time may account for the fact that when a child is admitted to care the overall priority accorded the case rapidly diminishes, the social worker feeling confident that at least the child is safe. Although few social workers made explicit reference to this, one who did put it in the following way.

> Something which quite often happens is that once the child is safe, one's interest falls off a bit. I suppose it is bound to happen — once a **91**

child is in care there is a bit of pushing to the middle of the pile rather than to the top.

Furthermore it was clear that in the period following admission to care, social workers can have some difficulty in determining who is the client. Whilst strictly speaking it is the child who is the client from this stage and thus the child's interests which are to be represented, social workers invariably tended to relate to the parents. For example, each of the following comments was drawn from cases where the child had been in care for more than a year and had infrequent and irregular contact with the parent(s).

I think we really need to give her (*mother*) another chance.

It can't have been easy for her (*mother*) — now that she's had a break, it's only fair that we try again.

I feel really sorry for them (*parents*) — they wouldn't deliberately do these kids any harm, they're devoted to them.

The combination of this and the relaxation in priority post-admission to care means that there can be a protracted delay in addressing the question of the *child's* future. Describing the effects this had had on the case she had just taken over, a social worker said:

I can see what's happened here. What we've been doing for years and years is to prop up this mother and we haven't even managed to maintain the situation. It's only got progressively worse. It's easy for me. I'm new to the case and I can see that we've really done nothing for this kid. It's not going to be easy at nine but hopefully I can find something for him better than what he's got — in another few years it would certainly just be hopeless.

The reactive planning process set in motion by this lull in activity undoubtedly reduced social workers' ability to subsequently plan. However the data suggest that in other respects the scope and activity of planning was constrained, thus compounding this situation.

Social workers' knowledge of the law

Social workers' increased willingness over the study period to consult a representative of the authority's legal department before admitting a child to care suggested that they appreciated that the law could usefully reinforce their actions in removing children from their families and prevent their return. There was however, little corresponding appreciation of the provisions of the law in relation to allowing children to leave the care system via adoption. For example, when asked in cases where it was clear that the child would not be returning home whether there were plans for adoption, social workers invariably replied: 'Yes that would be ideal but the parents would never agree to it'. Furthermore while social workers claimed that it was lack of parental consent to adoption which precluded adoption for 19 children under 11 years who had no or virtually no contact with their parents, it was apparent that they had not actually raised this matter with the parents. In this respect social workers assumed not only that the parents would object but, and more importantly in this context, that nothing could be done about this. In other words their lack of knowledge of the law in relation to adoption restricted the scope of what they felt it was possible to achieve for children, which in turn reinforced their tendency to focus on the in-care situation.

The risks of planning

The fact that planning entailed taking risks also served to deter social workers from planning. Broadly speaking it was felt that if by planning, children's interests were no more likely to be advanced than to suffer, then it was 'safer' to let events run their natural course.

Fear that planning would 'rock the boat' as far as the parents were concerned was particularly acute in cases where it was felt that given time, the parents would in any event opt out of children's lives. This was especially marked in cases which social workers described as those characterised by 'lingering parents', that is parents who maintained minimal contact with their children but gave no real indication that they would ever have them back. Since these parents would probably ultimately drop out of the situation themselves, planning that the child did not return home raised the possibility that the parents would be provoked into removing the child from care, and therefore planning was not undertaken.

However in other respects, it was clear that fear of provoking parents could itself lead to the 'lingering parent' situation and constrain social workers' ability to plan. Social workers tended to adopt an approach of passive discouragement and implicit obstruction towards parents whose intentions they were unsure of such that, for example, they were never explicitly denied access to their children but neither were they encouraged. It seemed likely that given support some families would have recognised that it was in their child's interests that he or she be relinquished. However the approach adopted by the social worker precluded this type of assistance to parents. In the absence of support, parents often lingered on the periphery of children's lives, being sufficient enough of a presence to children that alternative plans were limited in scope.

Planning, or at least making plans formally known, also increased the likelihood that the parents might take their complaints to court and social workers were not entirely confident that the courts would share their interpretation of a child's situation. For example, during the study period, a number of cases in our sample were involved in court situations where parents were successful in their challenge and the children were returned home, whilst in another, the case of a two-year-old who had already been in care for more than a year, the court adjourned the case for no less than six months in order that the mother might benefit from a period of assistance from the social worker. In each case, the social worker concerned had attempted to make and implement permanent plans for the child, in one case by adoption and in the others by placing the children in situations felt guaranteed to lead to adoption. Each of the social workers stated that they had 'lost' the court case because they had based their evidence on the 'best interest of the child' as opposed to presenting the parents as 'bad' parents. They felt that the court, on the other hand, looked solely at the fact that the parents were now saying they wanted the child back, and disregarded the fact that their previous care of the children had been poor and that the children had already been in care for some time. Furthermore, as a result of their experience, the social workers felt that the court took the view that parents were always entitled to try again and, as such, children's interest were a secondary consideration.

In this context, the significance of these decisions by the court is the impact they have, not just on the social workers directly involved, but on the perceptions of the role of the law in the wider social work community. In each of the above cases, the social workers had consciously attempted to avoid being in the situation where plans evolved, and had endeavoured positively to pursue a course of action in the child's interest. The experience suggested that the final authority, the court, did not support such an approach unconditionally. Thus, for these workers and their colleagues, the implications of the court's decision was that in pursuing an active approach, one ran a greater risk of harming the child's interest than one did by letting events run their natural course. As one of these social workers put it:

> There's no doubt about it — I'll play it safe in future. I am only prepared to get my hands burnt once.

Planning — whose responsibility?

Recognising that planning was risky, and hence stressful, a few of the study social workers had independently attempted to take positive countermeasures. For example, two social workers, both very experienced had agreed with their team leader that in order to communicate what were likely to be unpopular decisions to the parents, the team leader would accompany the social worker and actually relay the decision, thus freeing the social worker to assume a positive and supportive role towards the parents. Another social worker, again very experienced, attempted to ensure that decisions were not taken about parents' rights in relation to a child without there first being a meeting involving the area director, team leader and parents, and in any event insisted that parents were always made aware of such decisions in the form of a letter from the area director.

However, there was little evidence of support being routinely available to caseholders. Indeed the absence in each of the study areas of any formal mechanism to ensure meaningful planning and to monitor the progress of plans indicated that planning for children in care had little departmental priority. However this is not to say that social workers would not have welcomed more positive guidelines.

In several respects it was clear that social workers felt that the system in which they operated did not support the notion of purposeful planning and this in itself inhibited the extent to which they were prepared to expose themselves to the risks of planning. The following comments from social workers about their experiences of attempting to plan indicate what a negative experience they found this to be within their own departments:

It's all very well that I have to show initiative to make decisions but at the end of the day, this (*action recommended by social worker*) has to be blessed by someone up above. All that comes back is 'no, this can't be done'. Nobody ever tries to give you any other ideas though.

I don't know, its like being on a see-saw, this case, I've tried but the department is going to have to be a bit clearer here. They just nod their head to anything and anybody. They say 'yes' to me and at the same time say 'yes' to the parents. You have to have some support in making these early decisions.

I've tried it all ways — in this case I thought enough is enough and I stuck my neck out and said: I have a plan, what do you think? Nobody said 'yes', nobody said 'no', there is just nothing. I don't know what it all means. Nobody else seems worried — they seem quite happy to let it all drift on.

In other words, not only did departments not appear to give planning much priority in a formal sense, they offered individual social workers little support in attempting to fulfill the department's statutory responsibilities. The fact that many social workers' behaviour takes the form of 'satisficing' (Simon 1957), accepting situations which represent the minimum of what they think they should ideally be, may well be their way of coping with the situation in which they find themselves.

Summary

On the basis of looking at the plans stated by social workers and at what happens to children at various stages of children's care careers, it seems evident that children's futures are rarely dealt with in the synoptic manner suggested by the planning approach. Indeed the postponement of planning in the early stages of children's care careers often means that the activity of planning becomes subsequently constrained, children's futures being moulded by their prevailing circumstances and the vagaries of their in-care situation. In this process, social workers carrying cases appear as individuals whose behaviour is both passive and reactive. The chapter concluded in a description of aspects of the overall care system which seemed to inhibit social workers from adopting a more purposeful stance. Since the *modus operandi* of social workers will at least in part have been shaped by their own practical experience, it seems likely that any future attempts to promote planning will need to recognise the existence of organisational barriers to planning. hat any future attempts to promote planning will need to recognise the existence of organisational barriers to planning.

CHAPTER SEVEN
Vehicles for Decision-making and Planning

Recognising that there are three 'formal' contexts within which discussion of children's cases may take place in social services departments: statutory reviews, case conferences and supervision sessions, provision was made in the research design to assess the impact each of these had on planning and decision-making. Therefore, wherever possible and appropriate, we attended meetings held on the sample cases as well as discussing reviews, case conferences and supervision in the course of interviews with social workers. However the fact that, as researchers, we spent substantial periods of time in local area offices reading files and generally 'being around' meant that we were able to observe the often more informal discussions which took place in relation to children too. This chapter begins by considering each of the formal vehicles in turn, moves on to consider the more informal processes noted and concludes by discussing the relative contributions of both the formal and informal to planning and decision-making.

Reviews

Statutory reviews have been a feature of child care practice since they were introduced by the Children Act 1948. Since then, they have been widened to include an increasing range of children and to encompass an ever-increasing range of functions. Initially, reviews were required only for children in foster care and were designed primarily to ensure that the child was receiving adequate care and the placement was in no way detrimental to the child. As such, reviews were rather limited in scope, safeguarding rather than promoting the welfare of children.

With the *Boarding Out of Children Regulations* (1955), the frequency of the review and the areas it should cover were specified: the review was to be carried out after three months of placement and thereafter at intervals of no more than six months; and was to consider the health, welfare, conduct and progress of the child. The requirement to 'review' was extended to include all children in care, regardless of placement, by the Children and Young Persons Act 1969 and the same Act built in the additional requirement that '. . . if a care order is in force . . . to consider in the course of the review whether to make application for the discharge of the order'. Broadly speaking, the impact of these developments has been in structuring the format of reviews which appears to have been strongly influenced by the recommendations outlined in the 1955 Boarding Out Regulations. The purpose and value of reviews, however, became increasingly vague and open to variable interpretation.

For some time case review systems have been advocated in all fields of social work (see, for example, Goldberg and Warburton, 1979) with the dual aim of improving the monitoring capacity of social services departments and of improving the quality of work undertaken by social workers with their clients. In the child care field, Sinclair (1982) has pointed out that one of the effects of Rowe and Lambert's 'Children who Wait' study (1973) has been that reviews have been promoted as a way of monitoring not only the material care which children receive but also the planning undertaken by social services departments on behalf of their child clients. In this respect, the review was seen as a vehicle for the implementation of the Children Act 1975, which in Sections 3 and 59 placed a duty on local authorities 'to give first consideration to the need to safeguard and promote the welfare of the child in care throughout childhood' in reaching any decision concerning the child.

The clear implication for social work practice was the emphasis which the Act laid on the need for sound and careful planning in social work management, as opposed to providing immediate solutions to problems, without necessarily considering what the future should or was likely to hold for the child concerned.

The Act also recognised the lack of official guidelines on the form the review should take and in Schedule 3 it is stated, 'the Secretary of State may by regulations make provision as to (a) the manner in which cases are to be reviewed (b) the considerations to which the local authority have to have regarding reviewing cases . . . and (c) the time when a child's case is to be reviewed and the frequency of subsequent reviews . . .'.

Although such draft regulations were prepared by the Department of Health and Social Security during the course of the research, they were not formally issued due to the estimated costs involved. A study of the Boarding Out of Children carried out simultaneously with this piece of work by the Social Work Service of the Department of Health and Social

Security (1981) put forward, although without statutory force, the purpose of reviews as then seen by the department:

> The overall purpose of the review can be summarised as bringing knowledge of the past and present to bear on formulating plans for the child's future. In order to do so, it is necessary to bring together and consider all the aspects of parenting shared by the agency, and those caring for the child and by his natural parents. The review must take into account the views of the child and make use of the expertise of other professionals who are involved, for example in his health care and in education. The review can also provide an important opportunity for monitoring the work of the social worker who is responsible for ensuring that the child's needs are met. Plans may have to be made within the constraints of available resources but they should form the basis of future work with the child, his family and his carers and be related to well defined time scales. They need consideration both between and at subsequent reviews to ensure that they are amended as appropriate, that there is a commitment to them by those responsible for taking action, and that the required action is carried out. (page 13).

More recently still, the DHSS has circulated a consultative document on reviews (1984) which states:

> . . . the review is not, or not necessarily, the forum for decisions on a child's future . . ..

The procedures adopted to fulfill the statutory requirement

In the absence of clear official guidelines, other than the Boarding Out Regulations, the authorities in this study had developed a variety of review systems. In most, the basic review procedure clearly derived from the 1955 Boarding Out Regulations and had changed little in the intervening period whilst in a few, attempts had been made to modify the system to reflect current concerns in social work practice. What all had in common was some type of departmental review form and a system of reminders of the need for reviews.

The forms themselves varied considerably in length and content. For example, in one department, the review form consisted of a single page headed 'Summary of Progress' with sub-headings entitled 'Plans' and

'Senior's Comments'; while another department had a six-page review form, with more than 20 sub-headings. In some departments, one form was used for all children in care, whilst in others there were separate forms depending on whether the child was fostered, home on trial or in residential care. Interestingly despite the requirement to review the need for a care order when such an order was in force, none of the authorities involved had a distinct sub-heading for this topic. Furthermore with only one exception, none of the forms used had a separate sub-heading stating the reasons for the child currently being in care.

The procedure for completing the form also varied: usually, it was completed by a social worker and if a meeting was to take place, the social worker completed most of the form in advance; in others a 'reviewing officer', someone other than the social worker holding the case, completed the form in the course of the meeting, that is the business of the meeting was to complete the proforma; and in others someone, not necessarily the social worker, completed the review form after the meeting had been held. However, whilst one of the above might be described as an area's review procedure, elements of all three were found to exist in most areas. In all areas, a copy of the review form was placed on the child's file and this often proved to be the most informative piece of documentation in the file, this, however, being more a statement of the paucity of information in the rest of the file than an accolade to the review form. Apart from the fact that where new decisions or plans had been made, the review forms generally omitted both to record whether these had been reached in the course of the review and to explain the reasons for the change, the forms invariably contained inaccuracies. Whilst these inaccuracies were seldom of major significance to an individual child's case history, the fact that they were perpetuated in successive review forms, suggested that in their completion a routine approach was followed.

This routinisation was also evident in the procedure for scheduling reviews. With the exception of one area, the fact that the review was due was communicated to the social worker or the social worker's team leader by a member of the administrative staff, either from the department's headquarters or from within the area office. Such reminders were on the whole based on the date of the child's admission to care and six-monthly reminders thereafter, rather than on a knowledge of dates of actual reviews completed, and more importantly, regardless of the needs of the case. In two areas, carrying out reviews was seen as such a time-consuming exercise that systems had been devised to simplify matters: in one area, reviews were scheduled according to the initial letters of the child's surname and distributed throughout the year, whilst in another the children in care population was divided, such that half the children were reviewed in two named months of the year and the other half in a further two named months. In so organising reviews, little recognition was taken of the need to review boarded out children within three months of placement, far less of admission. Moreover, whilst we heard it said on a number of occasions that there was nothing to prevent an 'early' review being held, this was rarely encountered in practice, and it appeared that the systems devised to schedule reviews created the tendency for reviews to occur at minimum, rather than maximum, periods of six months.

Furthermore none of these systems included provision for checking that reviews did take place. In this respect, it is useful to note that whilst a minimum of 310 reviews was due on the 185 sample cases in the course of the study year, 196 were actually completed. On the whole reviews did tend to be completed on a fairly regular basis but as is apparent not necessarily at maximum intervals of six months. In addition it was clear that some cases go from year to year without being reviewed at all. For example, no review was carried out on 24 of the sample cases who remained in care throughout the year-long study period. In other words, a by-product of the attempt to ensure the fulfilment of the statutory requirement to review was the tendency to view the review as an administrative procedure with little, if any, professional purpose.

The review itself

Although it was said in seven of the eleven areas participating in the research that reviews always took the form of meetings, in practice the situation was rarely so straightforward and there was little evidence of a standard format of review meetings. On the other hand, in two of the four remaining authorities, where no such general statement was made, it was noted that on the whole the review was not deemed to have been completed until there had been some form of discussion, however brief. Overall, approximately two thirds of the reviews carried out on the study children in the course of the research period involved some form of meeting.

The 67 reviews which did not involve meetings were generally referred to as 'paper' reviews and tended to be concerned with particular groups of children: for example children well established in long-term foster care, particularly those placed with relatives (48), children placed home on trial (5) and young people held in penal establishments (4). In these circumstances the review entailed the child's social worker completing the departmental review form, which was then circulated at least to the social workers' team leader. Very occasionally discussions followed but this was generally purely for clarification of a point and the discussion, or a summary of it, was rarely recorded on a review form. In terms of decision making and planning such reviews served little function. Arguably, in a number of the cases involved, there was no need for planning and decision making and the main purpose served by completing the review form was to ensure that there was an up-to-date record of the child's particulars on file.

However to describe the remaining two-thirds (129) of reviews as 'meetings' is rather misleading, as they ranged from five-minute encounters between two people to hour-long events attended by more than ten people. As with the 'no meeting' reviews there were few discernible differences between areas or admission groups of children, but there were differences based on the child's placement.

For example, reviews of younger children in residential care were almost without exception meetings and, all in all, fairly major events: they took place in the residential establishment where the child was placed and those present included not only the social worker and team leader, but the child's immediate 'carers' and the head of the home, a representative from the child's school and possibly health and social work specialists. Moreover, this type of review tended to be chaired by a relatively senior member of staff who had no direct involvement with the child or family: for example, the director in charge of the area in which the residential unit was situated sometimes fulfilled this function.

At the other end of the spectrum, reviews of children in foster care tended to involve only two people, the social worker and one other. Over the period of the research, there was increasing discussion amongst social workers about the need to involve foster parents in the reviews of children in their care. Whilst there were some developments in this respect, such as providing foster parents with forms to complete prior to the review date, there were in fact very few instances of foster parents being involved in reviews by virtue of their attendance at a review meeting. In general, then, foster care reviews took the form of a discussion within the area office between two social services department employees, these invariably being the child's social worker and his/her team leader.

During the study period there were attempts in a couple of areas to replace team leaders with more 'neutral' reviewing officers who had no direct involvement with, or immediate line management responsibility for, the case. Sometimes the area director performed this function, sometimes an area child care specialist and sometimes another team leader within the office. It was clear, however, that 'neutral' reviewing officers were often uncomfortable in their role: 'other' team leaders, in particular, not wishing to challenge what was apparently occurring on a case with the blessing of the social worker's own team leader. Moreover, given that social workers had fairly limited contact with these reviewing officers, myths built up about what certain reviewing officers expected, how thorough they were etc.

In consequence social workers structured their presentation of information at reviews according to their perception of different reviewing officers. For example, with some it was felt better to reveal as few details of the case as possible and get the review over; with others it was known that the reviewing officer disapproved in general terms of certain courses of action so if a social worker wished to pursue a certain line, he or she would have embarked on this course prior to the review; whilst other reviewing officers it was believed would offer genuinely helpful suggestions.

In one respect, the social worker's scope and power to influence is again highlighted. However, notwithstanding this, 'neutral' reviewing officers sometimes left social workers feeling very unsupported, a feature commented on by a number of social workers and about which they were very bitter. They felt, and indeed we noted, that on occasions 'neutral' reviewing officers withdrew from situations where they were likely to become involved in making decisions which ran counter to the principles of child care, for example stating that since a child would not be returning home and was unsuitable for foster care, he or she would have to remain long-term in residential care. Features such as these served only to militate against the review fulfilling a positive role in relation to decision-making and planning, where indeed this was seen to be part of its function.

Perceptions of reviews

Although efforts were made to attend as many types of review meetings as possible, the researchers did not attempt to discuss systematically the review either before it took place or thereafter with anyone other than the social worker. Our comments then are largely restricted to social workers' perceptions, and where references to other participants' perceptions are made, these are obviously selective. It must also be acknowledged that during the period of research the review received increasing coverage in the social work literature not only as a forum for decision-making and planning but as a venue for the participation of the child, and also the parents (Page and Clark, 1977; Davis 1982).

Broadly speaking, those in the field rarely saw reviews as taking decisions or formulating plans but rather as part of an administrative procedure — a statutory requirement. Indeed, in some instances, it was quite apparent that the social worker was unaware of the legal responsibility to review, thinking it was a procedure of their own department. Some quotations are given to illustrate the overall impressions which emerged:

> Yes. There is a review due here — I'll just fill that form in.

> I'm hopeless at these bureaucratic things.

> There was a meeting but I wouldn't call it a discussion — I just told them what I was planning.

> I'd never have thought of making decisions at reviews — they just give the seal of approval to decisions that have already been made really.

> Yes, there will be a review but that will only be a five-minute affair.

> There was a review — that was a typical non-event.

Perceptions such as these were not necessarily confined to main grade social workers. At one review attended, comprising the social worker and a team leader from another team, the team leader read the review form completed by the social worker and then said to her: 'OK: I'll waffle something about . . . will that do?' and that concluded the review.

On another occasion, the researcher's presence in the office for the purpose of attending specific reviews was quite openly stated as being the only reason why the discussion had taken place. Despite the fact that a meeting had been scheduled, when it came to the day, the participants would have been happy to have only exchanged the review form.

Finally, one researcher was asked on a number of occasions why she wished to attend reviews when she was interested in decision-making. As one area director put it 'But reviews — they are about what's already happened — that's what the word means — re-view. I chair several reviews, and I've never allowed a review to make a decision — that's for the social worker and team leader, not for the review'.

To a considerable extent, social workers' perception of the purpose of the review will have been moulded by their own experience of how the review operates in practice. From the above, it would seem that decision-making and planning are not substantial components of reviews. The above comments also reflect the lack of authority associated with the review: in terms of outcome, this is quite significant and contrasts sharply with the authority and impact the case conference may have.

The case conference considers specific problems and concludes by recommending specific action. This recommendation is at least highly influential and social workers would feel they had to have a very good reason not to follow such a recommendation. The review does not hold such authority and hence its potential as a vehicle for direct planning is likely to be impaired. The outcome of the reviews is considered in greater detail after examining participation in the review process and the content of the review.

Participants in reviews

During the period of the research and subsequently, there has been a great deal of discussion in the social work journals about the rights of various individuals to be party to a review, the argument being in the case of the child, for example, that since the review is making a decision or planning for that child, he or she, if old enough, should be involved in that process (see for example Page and Clark 1977). However in such discussions of 'involvement', the distinction is rarely made between attendance, participation and consultation.

Of the 129 reviews described as meetings, children (generally teenagers) were present in seven cases, natural parents not at all and in nine cases at least one foster parent attended. In our experience, then, it was unusual for the child or either of the biological or foster parents to be present at a review although it should be said that social workers increasingly indicated that they felt foster parents and children should be invited to attend. The lack of colleague status ascribed to foster parents was apparent in that, in contrast, residential workers were generally present at reviews if the child was placed in residential care.

To comment on consultation is more difficult as consultation does not necessarily imply participation by attendance. Where a participant did not attend, the process of consultation was likely to be undertaken by the social worker. However, there was little evidence of any distinguishable procedure for ensuring consultation.

In a few local authorities, the review form had a sub-section 'Child's View' an in others, it was the practice to send a letter to the foster parents informing them that a review would be taking place and enclosing a specially designed form for their comments, should they wish to contribute. However, these practices were not typical and there was no evidence of any formal corresponding effort to consult biological parents.

In considering the question of participation in the review process, one has also to pose the question 'participation in what?' thus raising again the overall function of the review.

The experience of the research team suggests that the primary function served by the attendance of foster parents, biological parents or child in such a setting was the passing of information, particularly passing information to social services staff. Whilst such information might then, or subsequently, be used in taking a decision, the exchange *per se* did not take the form of participation in decision-making or planning. Indeed this was often a source of antagonism, particularly with biological parents and adolescents who believed that being asked to state what they felt should happen was tantamount to saying this was what would happen.

Lack of agreement on the purpose of the review and/or on the status of the residential worker in planning and decision-making was also a source of friction. However, because residential workers were at the same time both present at reviews and key holders of a valuable resource, the placement, their participation in the review and potential ability to influence events was significantly greater than that of other participants. In a sense, they could force the need to make a decision.

When neither child nor foster parent attended the review, social workers did generally make some attempt to have contact with the foster parents at least prior to the review. Such contacts, however, did not appear to be any different from other 'routine' contact and were of the form of 'keeping in touch', or 'keeping up-to-date', i.e. information was again passing to social workers about children.

It was particularly noted that there was little evidence to suggest that social workers actively sought specific information from foster parents. For example, it was clear from what later happened in some cases that the foster parents were (or were not) interested in adopting the child, yet this issue was not raised within the review process.

As far as the child's biological parents were concerned, our limited data suggest that contact was unlikely to occur because of an impending review, and in any event decreased the longer a child was in care and was most likely to relate to the parents' own physical and material circumstances, rather than to the child's situation or directly on how the one might bear on the other.

It is quite clear, then, that attendance at a review is not necessarily equivalent to participation in the review process. Similarly, one might query the appropriateness of the term 'consultation': consultation implies that some consideration is being given to the possibility of change or to the establishment of a new status, whereas the exchanges involved in the review process do not indicate such a starting point but appear to be concerned with describing a current situation. Whilst the review's focus on the current situation is probably attributable to its historical origins this nonetheless indicates that, in practice, the primary purpose of the review is not seen as being the formulation of plans or the taking of decisions.

The involvement of other key persons in the review process has also been recommended. In this respect, much obviously depends on the circumstances of individual cases but where children of school age are concerned, the involvement of teachers has been identified as being of importance. Once again this tended to depend on whether the child was in foster or residential care. In the latter instance, it appeared to be standard practice to invite a representative of the school to a review, and although such invitations were not always accepted, schools did tend to submit written reports for reviews. This was not so for the child in foster care other than where there was an already identified education problem, in which case it would be reported by the social worker.

Otherwise, it was unusual for outside specialists to be involved at a review meeting, although where they were active in a case, mention of this was made. That they appeared to be more likely to be invited to attend case conferences is again indicative that the review is not seen as a forum for taking decisions.

Finally, reference must also be made to the presence of departmental specialists in review meetings. This generally only occurred in reviews concerning children in residential care and normally involved an officer with overall responsibility for residential resources. As such, these officers were concerned with the use being made of the placement rather than with the child or his needs. However, in one area it was noted that the area fostering officer was attempting to be regularly involved in reviews, and particularly those of children in residential establishments. This was an action taken at the initiative of the individual concerned and he felt that departmental commitment to it was low and that his colleagues preferred him to attend only by invitation.

The content of the review

As will be apparent from what has been said so far, there is no single model which covers all the types of review encountered in the study areas. Furthermore, the relevance of different information and the detail in which it needs to be presented will be largely determined by the circumstances of the individual case and the stage at which it is discussed. Here, we are concerned to examine the more general focus of the review and to relate this to the review's *potential* role in relation to decision making and planning. In this respect, analysis of the data collected by attending reviews suggests that their overall focus is on the past and present rather than the future.

It was noted that the question 'Why is the child in care?' was rarely addressed either on the review form or directly in the course of discussion. On the other hand, the reasons for the child's admission and the circumstances surrounding it (not necessarily the same as why the child is currently in care) did tend to be recorded on the review form and often featured to a substantial degree in discussion. The inclusion of past circumstances and the exclusion of current circumstances suggests that, as far as social workers are concerned, it is the past which is important. By not giving direct consideration to the child's current circumstances in this way, it is unlikely that purposeful plans can be made on the child's behalf.

The emphasis on the circumstances of admission arose from the tendency to use this topic as an introduction to the review proper: it served as an *aide-memoire* for participants to the review (particularly those not directly involved with the case) and 'got the ball rolling'. Nonetheless, having established this line of discussion, it appeared very difficult to move on to another footing. Therefore, what appeared to occur was that in describing the circumstances of admission, the circumstances of the parents were covered, with the result that the next topic following automatically was the current circumstances of the parent.

An analysis of topics covered in the review indicated that this aspect —

the parents' current situation — occurred more consistently than any other. Reviews where it did not feature accounted for less than five per cent of the total. Furthermore, this happened regardless of whether parents were in contact with the child, or whether future plans incorporated parental involvement, as is indicated in the following example:

> In the review of a six-year-old-boy, who had been fostered with the same couple from birth and was now placed with them on a long-term basis, the review began by those present reading the previously circulated review form. Having done this, the reviewing officer asked to be reminded why the child had been admitted to care in the first place. This, and the fact that there had been no parental contact for more than three years, having been outlined, the reviewing officer then commented that he recalled the case and proceeded to recount his own recollections, finally asking what the parents were now doing. The social worker outlined the parental situation as she currently understood it — having had no personal contact herself.
>
> The reviewing officer then stated — 'and I understand from what you say that the child is quite settled with Mr and Mrs Y' Having had this confirmed, the reviewing officer commented that he, like the social worker, felt it quite appropriate for the placement to continue.

This example illustrates the extent to which consideration of the past and the parents' current situation may occupy a substantial proportion of the overall review period. Whilst one might view much of such discussion as describing the child's family background it did not constitute a comprehensive social history of the child, nor was it directly related to how the future would or should develop.

Analysis of the topics covered in reviews also shows that reference is generally made to the suitability of the child's placement. Nonetheless, the manner in which this was covered did not indicate that the review was thought of as an aid to decision-making and planning: for example, where no major problems were identified or reported for the child in a particular foster placement, it was assumed the placement was appropriate and no further consideration was given to how it might be developed in the future. In other words, the review was concerned with the current suitability of the placement rather than with the suitability of the current placement.

Where the child was placed in residential care, this differed only to the extent that, depending largely on the age of the child, fostering could be seen as a more appropriate placement. Thus, whilst reviews gave consideration to the question of placement, there was a tendency to approach the topic in a routine manner and with little direct reference to the needs of the individual child or to how these needs might change with time.

Some importance might also be attached to the fact that alongside the emphasis on the current suitability of placement, consideration was only infrequently given in reviews to examining the direct work being undertaken by the social worker with the child, parent and/or caretaker, either currently or that deemed appropriate to the future. This omission is further indicative of the review's function in practice. The emphasis on placement suggests that the review may have more in common with the model of the *Boarding Out Regulations* than it has with the model advocating the review as a forum for planning.

Finally a further feature of the content of reviews was the degree to which the topic of adoption was, in fact, avoided. Although there were instances where adoption was discussed, the topic was generally initiated by a foster parent who wished to adopt (see also Chapter Six).

More often, the subject was not directly addressed at all even though raising it might, at least, have served the purpose of discounting it. For example a review was attended where the social worker had previously described the foster parents and child as eminently suited for adoption. However although the foster parents were present at the review, the topic of adoption was not raised and on the form where the question 'Is adoption appropriate?' was asked, a negative response was given.

The above example indicates the tendency within reviews to avoid looking forward and to fail to consider any alternatives to care itself. Commonly, the review becomes pre-occupied with the past and with the current situation and this is unlikely to be conducive to the development of a planning or decision-making function. There were only few exceptions to this and these are taken up in looking at the outcomes of reviews.

Outcomes of reviews

On the basis of the discussion so far, it is apparent that reviews are not perceived as taking decisions and do not function in an explicitly decision-making manner. Their overall effect, then, in terms of outcome is to endorse what is currently happening on a case. In this sense this means that they reinforce the plan or approach already being followed.

In Care

Looking at the outcomes of reviews does, however, yield two further useful insights into the nature of planning and decision-making in child care.

First, although individual reviews rarely directly fulfilled a planning or decision-making function, by looking at cases over time, it is apparent that reviews may contribute to planning and decision-making in a less direct and generally unrecognised manner. For example in considering only the present and immediate future, reviews typically concluded by confirming that the current placement should continue. A corollary of this was that no other placement should be looked for and this could have the effect of not encouraging return home, but of maintaining the current situation, that of remaining in care. The following cases illustrates this point:

Donald

Donald was admitted to care suffering from hypothermia when he was only a few months old. A care order was obtained and he was placed in a foster home.

At the first review, the social worker wrote: 'Donald is now eight months old and although it is slow, progress is maintained. There is no reason to consider any change'. No further comments were added as a result of the review.

At the next review, approximately six months later, the social worker wrote: 'A steady, normal and happy development as far as Donald is concerned. He is a very lively child who demands a fair degree of control. His mother sees him almost every week. No reason to consider any change'. At the third review the social worker wrote 'Donald continues to make good normal progress. He mixes well with other children and is secure in the home; he gets a lot of care from his loving foster parents. Mother's situation continues to deteriorate, she is now pregnant and does not know the child's father. The care of (an older child) is still the subject of concern; nursery school are keeping a watchful eye. She has not visited Donald for almost a month. No change envisaged'.

Each of these review forms was counter-signed by the reviewing officer and no comment was made about the future other than 'Placement to continue'. This comment was repeated in subsequent reviews until at a review when the child was almost five, the report stated: 'Mr and Mrs (foster parents) have said that if it is possible they would like to continue to look after Donald' and at a later stage it was added 'No change envisaged'.

Gerald

Gerald was admitted to care at his mother's request when he was 18 months old. Whilst he was expected to return home, it was said that this was unlikely to be before he started school. This was reflected in review forms in the statement 'Placement to continue in the meantime'.

Gerald was three-and-a-half at the start of the research, and the last review on file stated: 'There have been no disruptive parental visits. Gerald seems secure in his placement. As it is now unlikely that he will have a stable home background, it was heartening to hear Mr and Mrs (foster parents) are now talking of Gerald's home being with them when he leaves school, and afterwards if he wishes'.

At the next review, the social worker reported that the foster parents had formally applied to become long-term foster parents to Gerald and that he felt this application should be supported. No direct reference was made to the change in 'plan' but in the subsequent research interview, the social worker said 'I think it's been implicit for some time that he was making such progress in the foster home, he was likely to remain there. The foster parents have said that they are keen on this and it was formalised at the review last week.'

Cases such as these demonstrate that although decisions may not be taken directly at reviews, reviews may nonetheless play an influential role in the decision-making process. By taking little into account other than the child's current placement, such reviews did not encourage the social worker to consider alternatives. Thus, in such reviews if the placement was not presenting any obvious problems, the child remained in the placement and consequently in care. This, however, was only one aspect of the decision actually taken: the other, less recognised, being that the child would not return home. In other words, reviews may both contribute to decisions being taken by default and re-inforce a pattern of reactive planning.

Secondly, examining the outcome of individual reviews once more points up the strategic significance of the social worker holding the case. No matter what the type of review — paper review, brief discussion between team leader and social worker or full-scale discussion, the case holder was required to make a statement fairly early on in the proceedings about, at least, the immediate future for the child. These statements, generally written on the review form, defined the limits of the review.

For example, an analysis of the first 100 reviews in the study period showed that the main recommendations made by case holders were as follows: placement to continue (46), to continue search for alternative placement (13), to work towards child's return home (9), alternative placement to be sought or likely to be required in near future (no specifications) (9), to consider discharge of care order (6), alternative placement to be sought (type specified) (5), to consider possibility of home on trial (5) and other (7).

These recommendations were endorsed without any addition or revision in more than 90 per cent of the reviews and in the remainder, revisions were slight. For example, in some of the seven 'other' recommendations the social worker outlined a number of alternatives and stated that the purpose of the review was to consider the alternatives. In these reviews some of the alternatives might be eliminated or others added. Otherwise revisions to social workers' recommendations involved making more specific recommendations regarding the type of placement desirable. Moreover, in the few instances overall where the case holder attempted to open up the question of the child's future, the outcome of the review was rarely a definite conclusion but a list of alternatives (often extended by the social worker in the first place) which needed to be explored.

In other words, within the structure of the review, the initiative was left to the social worker to define the future and to raise, or not, the possibility of change.

Case conferences

Although procedures have been set out on a nationwide basis for the conduct of case conferences, these apply to the very specific situation where children are known to be or are suspected of being subject to non-accidental injury. In practice, however, the term 'case conference' is used in social service departments to refer to meetings of widely differing forms.

In the research period detailed information was collected on approximately 90 meetings which were referred to as case conferences and for convenience sake they are discussed here under the headings: inter-agency case conferences (approximating half the total), intra-agency case conferences (approximating one-third of the total) and assessment case conferences (the remainder.)

Inter-agency case conferences (47)

As the name implies, participants in these meetings included people from outside the social services department. The scale of these meetings, however, varied dramatically. At one end of the spectrum were the fairly informal chats between social worker, foster parents and residential staff and the child's teacher whilst at the other were the very formal case conference meetings which included representatives from the social services department, and senior representatives from the health and education services as well as the police.

In general, the latter type of conference was held in relation to children who in the past had been, or were believed to have been, subject to non-accidental injury. However other situations could also give rise to large scale inter-agency case conferences. For example, in the study period conferences were called where the implications of parents' serious mental illness had to be discussed and where there was a joint responsiblity for the child's placement such as where a child was placed in a special boarding school or an adolescent psychiatric unit.

Service to the family admissions were rarely the subject of such case conferences other than where some dramatic new development occurred on the case.

The purpose of these formal inter-agency case conferences was generally described by the social worker as two-fold: 'to exchange information' and 'to explore possibilities for the future'. The outcomes, however, were not necessarily as clearly defined. As with reviews, the same word was used to mean different things and different words were used to mean the same thing — for example, 'it was felt that . . .', 'the conference recommendation was that . . .', 'it was agreed . . .', 'we decided . . .'.

Certainly, at one conference we attended, the social worker left intending to do quite the opposite to that which was recorded as the decision of the conference by the chairman. The social worker said: 'It's only a case conference recommendation — I called the conference to see what they thought — I can take or leave their advice — because I called the conference doesn't mean I abdicate responsibility for taking decisions myself'. This was, however, a minority view and most workers felt that case conference recommendations carried weight.

The recommendations of such conferences were generally transmitted into action and could therefore be described as 'decision-making'. Furthermore, their influence was not confined to the social worker, the case holder. Indeed, social workers often called these conferences because of their influence on other parties to the case: a case conference recommendation could secure the release of desired placement resources, not only those controlled by the social services department but also, and in particular, those of the education department.

Whilst the composition of these large conferences varied, the underlying theme was that someone other than the social worker or team of representatives from the social services department was 'expert', either in child development in general or in relation to the particular child under discussion. Social workers, but also team leaders when present, adopted a low profile within the case conference meeting itself, making few if any, verbal contributions other than when invited to do so. They seemed especially to defer to members of the medical profession — paediatricians, child psychiatrists — and to a lesser extent educational psychologists who on the basis of their assessment of the child drew conclusions about future placement, without necessarily being fully aware of the range of resources available.

Thus whilst social workers might query the validity of a recommendation in interview with us later, at the time of the conference they felt powerless to do so. In some circumstances, social workers got around this by subsequently claiming a change in the situation, but in others it was quite apparent that it was felt safer to follow the 'expert'. The case of Joseph illustrates the variable interpretation of the authority of a case conference recommendation.

Joseph

In the course of a routine medical examination, the paediatrician found evidence of bruising on 18-month-old Joseph. As a result, the paediatrician informed Joseph's parents that he would have to be detained in hospital. They refused to allow this and the paediatrician then telephoned the social worker informing her that a place of safety order was required since Joseph was bruised, suffering from malnutrition and should therefore on no account be allowed to return to his parents.

The social worker visited the hospital and managed to obtain the parents approval to voluntary care. The social worker was relieved that no more drastic measures had been necessary; the paediatrician was happy that Joseph was not returning home; and his parents accepted his need for hospital treatment and agreed to his being in care whilst this was required.

Because of the nature of Joseph's injuries, a case conference was automatically called, as it happened, on the same day that Joseph was due to be discharged from hospital. His parents made it clear that they expected him to return home. At the case conference the paediatrician was insistent that Joseph should not return home and demanded that a place of safety order should now be taken to ensure this. The paediatrician actually left the conference before it ended, but the minutes recorded: 'Recommendation: the Social Services Department should give serious consideration to taking care proceedings'.

The social worker left the conference and went straight to the home of Joseph's parents. She emphasised to them that she felt he should return home but thought this should be done gradually. Eventually, she managed to persuade the parents to agree to leave Joseph in care meantime and set about devising an elaborate plan to facilitate his return home. Explaining why she did not progress with care proceedings, the social worker later said in interview, 'I don't see why I should go for care proceedings — that whole thing was about the parents saying that they wanted Joseph back, and he wasn't to stay in care. I managed to reassure them that it would only be for a short time. I didn't really go against the case conference recommendation — it was just that I felt the conference was unnecessarily 'heavy'. What I've done has had the same effect'.

A few months later Joseph was discharged from care and all appeared at first to go well. Then there was renewed evidence of some slight neglect, and the parents began to avoid the social worker whereas they had previously been very co-operative. The social worker, fearing that there was a deterioration, called another case conference.

Explaining to the researcher why she did this, she said: 'Well, I still believe that this family could exist together. It would be hard work for us and wouldn't be what everyone would call an ideal family. But I've stuck my neck out already and feel that something may be about to go wrong now — nothing dramatic, I don't think but I'd like the conference to say what should happen — not me. It's not their endorsement I'm looking for. I'm not putting forward any arguments . . . it's their decision this time'.

In the smaller case conferences, the potential for conflict was much less apparent. Indeed, the calling of such a conference, usually by the social worker, was indicative of an already known consensus view. The actual conference served to formalise this and to agree a strategy. As one worker put it:

> I think we all knew the outcome in advance: it was just a question of ensuring everyone knew what their part was.

Whilst the issues discussed in these meetings were important to the child's well-being, they were not of the same dimension as those in more formal meetings. Likewise the social worker's role in relation to the two types of meeting differed: if not binding, the recommendations of large scale case conferences carried some weight whereas in the smaller less formal case conferences, the social worker tended to be a co-ordinator with the authority to change or amend the basic agreement without necessarily consulting the others concerned or recalling the conference.

As such then, these conferences were not truly decision-making but instruments which the social worker might use in the implementation of an overall plan or decision that had already been agreed. The subjects of these conferences tended to be children who had already been in care for some considerable time.

Children and parents were rarely directly involved in either of these types of conference. Where a more formal conference concerned a younger child, parents were generally aware that a meeting was to be held, having been informed by the social worker, and were also advised of the outcome, again by the social worker, because it most likely would have a direct bearing on their future role with the child. Therefore, although the calling of the conference did not permit them to put forward their own viewpoint, it did ensure that they were aware of decisions that had been made, and enabled them to respond if they so wished. In so far as the child was concerned, the results of decisions might eventually become very apparent but were not necessarily any more directly communicated.

Intra-agency case conferences (26)

Grouped together here are meetings which were described by social workers as conferences but were neither inter-agency conferences nor assessment case conferences. Broadly speaking they all entailed meetings between the fieldworkers and staff from the residential sector, which were called at the initiative of the residential sector.

Approximately half were characterised by a history of conflict between the social worker and the staff of the residential establishment where the child was placed such that, asked about the purpose of such conferences, social workers replied by describing a background of 'demands' made by the residential staff. These 'demands' related to the residential workers belief that the placement was inappropriate either because the child was disruptive within that home or because they felt that the child was 'drifting' unnecessarily in residential care. Frequently, then, the conference was held amid an atmosphere of tension and invariably took place because the residential staff had complained to a member of senior management.

In terms of outcome, these conferences were generally inconclusive and represented some form of temporary compromise. Whilst in this sense they were not necessarily 'decision-making', they did appear to affect subsequent action. For example, there was a number of instances where although it was not decided that the child would be moved (nor that he or she would remain), the child did subsequently move. Explaining this later social workers would speak of the atmosphere of the home not being conducive to the child's welfare. In this sense, examination of these conferences says more about the influence and power of residential staff and how field social workers react to this, than it does of the decision-making power of the conference itself. Children and parents were rarely involved in these conferences.

However, not all case conferences in this group were characterised by tension between the fieldwork and residential sectors. Whilst still initiated by staff of residential establishments, generally on a regular basis, the remaining meetings represented an opportunity to exchange information and discuss the future. Almost exclusively, they concerned adolescents in community schools and although the meetings were consistently described to us as case conferences, they appeared to have more in common with reviews: they were held at set intervals, sometimes being called post-admission meetings, and did not seem to be as problem-focused as other case conferences. They were concerned with case management within a placement or occasionally with plans for supporting the child after he or she left care.

Again these meeting rarely took decisions but they did appear to clarify the path of future directions. Similarly, it was rare for parents to be involved or even to be informed of such meetings but efforts were made to include children. Most commonly this took the form of inviting the young person in towards the end of a meeting. Since admission was not compulsory for the young person, one must conclude from their attendance that they found it worthwhile. Only rarely did they attend the whole of the conference, although in a number of instances they were invited to do so.

Assessment case conferences (17)

Reference has already been made in Chapter Four to the role of assessment case conferences at the time of admission to care. In general such meetings occurred in the early stages of children's care careers and without exception concerned older children. In some instances, assessment reports, and therefore a period in an observation and assessment centre, were requested by a court, whilst in others assessment followed the social worker's own decision to place a child in such an establishment. In the latter instance, the purpose of the conference was described by the social worker in wide terms:

> We have to decide what's to happen in the future.
> I've made no plans so far — that will happen at the conference.

However, by whatever route the young person came to be the subject of an assessment case conference, it was clearly expected that the outcome would be a decision or decisions. In practice, such was the outcome but on the whole the decisions were restricted to the child's future placement. The decision, too, was not so much that of the conference but of the assessment team staff who, although said to be making a recommendation, had often already taken steps to implement this by arranging an interview at an establishment for the child, and sometimes even securing placement before the conference meeting.

Again too, as in the formal inter-agency case conferences, social workers' reluctance to argue against the recommendation was noted, even although they might be less than happy with it. As has already been mentioned in Chapter Four, social workers appeared to be content to be absolved of the responsibility for making such decisions.

The notion of 'the expert' was evident again, and often openly acknowledged, not in the sense that the assessment team members were considered to be experts in a particular child or young person, or even in child development in general, but in the sense that such staff held detailed knowledge about a range of different resources. This expertise was largely confined to knowledge of residential resources but included not only information on the existence of these but on the type of regime and whether, for example, an establishment was vocationally orientated.

In effect, where assessment centre staff made a recommendation to the conference on the basis of such knowledge, this was accepted by the social worker, and the assessment centre staff then proceeded to attempt to implement it, the final decision being that of the recommended residential establishment to accept or reject the young person. Where such applications were unsuccessful, the conference was unlikely to be reconvened, but the social worker would be consulted and the centre staff would continue to negotiate the details of a move.

Direct participation in the conference also varied. In addition to the social worker, and the staff of the centre, an educational psychologist, psychiatrist and representatives from the child's school in the community might attend, but they might equally well only submit reports.

We found no marked trend in respect of attendance by parents and children within individual authorities or individual assessment centres, but on occasions parents were invited and did attend the whole of the conference. Where they did not, the decision of the conference was usually conveyed to them shortly afterwards by the social worker.

On the basis of a limited number of cases, it appeared to be rare for young people to attend these conferences in full, although on occasions they were invited in towards the end and told of the decision. Having been present in assessment centres for the purpose of attending case conferences, it became quite apparent that the young people in these establishments were well aware that meetings were being held which might have considerable implications for their future and they generally anxiously awaited news of the conference outcome.

These, then, were the main case conference types encountered in the research. All tended to influence decision-making, though not every one was intended to be a decision-making forum. More importantly, perhaps, they point up again the significance of the social worker as the individual who accepts or rejects recommendations for action and decides explicitly or otherwise what will actually occur. The extent to which other participants to case conferences play a significant role in decision-making is largely a reflection of the extent to which social workers allow them the scope to do so.

Supervision

Although the procedures outlined so far highlight the significance of the individual social worker, the fact must not be overlooked that each case holder is a member of a social work team, which is headed by a team leader or senior social worker, whose formal duties include staff supervision.

The term staff supervision has many meanings. In our understanding, the concept encompasses notions of staff development and training and the fact that time is set aside on a regular basis to allow this is indicative of the importance ascribed to such notions. In this sense, supervision has an 'enabling' function. However the fact that social workers state that they have a supervision session once a week or once a fortnight is not to say that they share anything approximating the same experience. For many, supervision is simply a monitoring function, particularly of the more administrative aspects of their work, such as the frequency of their visits, the completion of their case records etc. It therefore comes as a welcome relief to them if the sessions do not occur at the prescribed intervals and as long as their senior is available for consultation from time to time, they are quite content not to have 'supervision.'

On the basis of the study cases, supervision sessions did not occur at the departmentally prescribed frequency and, overall, their content was based on a narrow interpretation of 'supervision'. Generally speaking supervision operated in such a way that it acted primarily as a systematised consultation session. Time permitting, it served two basic functions: keeping the team leader up to date with difficult cases, and reminding social workers of the procedural requirements of certain steps.

Thus, a typical supervision session might begin by the team leader enquiring what was now happening on a certain case, that case being one which had recently demanded a considerable amount of time from the social worker. If the social worker indicated that the crisis had then subsided, the team leader left the matter; where the crisis continued, the team leader would be brought up to date with events and informed of any action the social worker had taken since the last discussion or intended to take in the near future. Beyond this, discussion or the relative merits of steps the social worker might be considering were left to the social worker to raise.

After running through such crisis cases, it was then left to the social worker to raise any points, he or she wished to discuss, and these generally concerned the more recent or impending crises. Should the team leader enquire of a case which was not currently demanding a lot of attention, the social worker terminated the discussion by stating: 'Everything is quiet there', or 'No that seems to be going OK'.

In other words, supervision sessions tended to be structured to deal with crisis-orientated work and were dependent on social workers raising issues. This is not to say that decisions were not taken in supervision sessions but that they were rarely described as such and generally took the form of endorsing what the social worker was already intending to do and not necessarily exploring other alternatives in the process. The following extract from one interview illustrates these points.

> *Social worker:* I discussed it in supervision with my team leader one day and we agreed that I should contact the fostering officer for a placement.

> *Researcher:* Do you mean the decision to pursue long-term fostering was taken by you and your senior at supervision?

> *Social worker:* No that's not strictly true. I had been thinking about it for sometime and I just happened to mention it to her. She thought it was a good idea. As it is, that was three weeks ago and I haven't had time to do anything about it. On the other hand, I might just as well have spoken to the fostering officer three weeks before that supervision session. I don't need to get my supervisor's permission for it. I will get down to it eventually, though. In that sense, I've made a decision about what will happen.

Perhaps even more importantly, there was no evidence that planning for children was a function of supervision and indeed the crisis-orientated focus of supervision sessions largely precluded this. In other words the initiative for planning rested with the social worker who received little direct departmental support unless it was directly raised by the worker in the supervision session.

Other vehicles for discussing cases

In the course of following the 185 sampled cases, it was clear that the discussion of cases was not confined to these formal settings. Meetings of other kinds took place to discuss child care cases and in addition child care cases invariably formed the focal point of informal office exchanges between social work colleagues. The significance of these in relation to the overall planning and decision-making process is discussed.

Procedures for 'quality control'

In three of the study offices, attempts were made to monitor and control the pattern of placement use by setting up what were generally referred to by social work managers as arrangements for quality control. Thus in each of these three offices there was some form of fostering panel to which social workers were expected to submit any plans they had for placing children in long-term foster care and in two there were structures designed to monitor the use of residential care, and the movement of children on care orders to placement home on trial.

Initial examination suggested that the existence of these arrangements would encroach on social workers' autonomy in decision-making and planning. However, since the scope of these arrangements was confined to considering specific proposals at certain times, their impact on decision-making and certainly on the development of plans for individual children was circumscribed.

Indeed, as a number of managers themselves commented, the manner in which these arrangements operated meant that the committee, panel or individual who was given the function of granting final approval invariably had no option other than to approve since the proposals were, in effect, already in the process of implementation. This was particularly marked where consideration was being given to placing a child with long-term foster parents or to returning a child home on a trial basis, since the social worker would not bring the matter forward for approval until such time as he or she was confident that it was appropriate and in this process was likely to have taken advanced steps in the direction of the proposal.

Thus in presenting the case for approval, a positive response was virtually guaranteed. In other words, although this type of arrangement assisted managers in managing resources, overall the management of individual cases was retained by the social workers dealing with the case.

Explicitly supportive meetings

This term has been reserved for meetings which were encountered in only two authorities. The principle underlying these was that social workers should not have to take difficult child care decisions alone and therefore, if a social worker wished, he or she could refer a case to a panel of professional experts and elected members for their support and advice.

It must be stressed that social workers were under no obligation to refer cases but the procedure served as a mechanism to help ensure that difficult decisions were taken and not avoided to the detriment of the child. This arrangement was used in only one sample case and there, the social worker felt that it would be appropriate to terminate parental access to the child, and indeed the social worker concerned certainly found it reassuring to have the group's backing.

However, over the study period these meetings fell in the favour of senior managers who felt that they were being mistakenly viewed by participating councillors and were consequently rather counter-productive. There were, at that time, no plans for substitutes or replacements embodying the same overall principle but precluding members of the council and the potential for political interference in individual cases.

Meetings with fostering and adoption specialists

Although the incidence of these meetings was not frequent amongst the sample cases, they have been included here because of their potential to impact on the general process of planning. In general such meetings were arranged at the request of social workers seeking guidance on what to do with a case and they described the purpose of the meeting in the following way:

> It is a tricky situation — I wondered if he (fostering specialist) could offer any advice on how to handle it.

> I'm not sure about this child. I wondered if he was a likely candidate for fostering.

However the outcomes of such meetings were rarely confined to the making of a decision. More commonly a consequence of the discussion was that the social worker would share the management of the case with the fostering or adoption officer who was both an 'expert' and a resource holder.

The experience of sharing the management of a case was one which social workers commented on very favourably such that, even although a child's placement might ultimately prove to be unsuccessful, their enthusiasm about the experience was scarcely affected. This may well be worth noting because such exchanges were generally characterised by

125

features not always evident in other aspects of decision-making and planning: they were generally time-limited and aimed at achieving a specific goal; involved drafting a plan of action with someone considered a peer but acknowledged as an expert; and throughout involved a clear definition of roles, accompanied by frequent exchanges of information.

Furthermore although these meetings themselves did not directly involve the child as participant, in content they focused to a considerable degree on the nature of what direct work with the child was necessary.

The impact of more informal discussions

In the context of considering the extent to which various means of 'discussing' cases contribute to decision-making and planning in child care, it would be highly remiss to ignore the influence of informal office exchanges.

Like Satyamurti (1981) we noted that the amount of time consumed in 'chatting' about cases was considerable. Social workers returned from visits or attempted visits to clients, to relay to whoever was around what had transpired. Similarly social workers bored by the paperwork with which they were occupied invariably attempted to relieve their boredom by engaging nearby colleagues in discussion of the intricacies of the case they were writing about. Team leaders, as well as others, passing through the office would stop to join these groupings. In this way, not only were individual cases discussed but general standards of practice were developed.

There were both positive and negative aspects to this. On the positive side, one social worker's experience of successfully attempting to do something could serve to suppport others to attempt, or at least consider, doing the same. In one office, for example, it was clearly believed that advertising for foster parents was 'a waste of time'. However, once it became common knowledge that one social worker had done this successfully, others folowed suit, deriving what guidance they could from their colleague in the process. On the other hand, a colleague's negative experience could serve to relegate certain steps to beyond what was generally regarded as an acceptable standard of practice.

In other words, given the limited impact on planning and decision-making of the more formal vehicles by which cases are discussed in social services departments, the reactive planning process described in the previous chapter may be a reflection of what has come to be defined by the group as an appropriate response to the anxiety-provoking and stressful situations with which group members have on an individual basis to deal.

Summary

Examination of reviews, case conferences and supervision sessions suggests that the impact of each on the social worker with case responsibility is limited. Although the arrangements for statutory reviews varied between authorities, we found overall that reviews were carried out in a perfunctory fashion. One-third of reviews were form-filling activities only and involved no discussion with other staff, parents or children. And even when review meetings were held, they tended to be regarded as routine and administrative in nature, focusing on what had happened in the past and on the current circumstances of the case. Few were problem-focused or involved forward planning.

Although case conferences usually had a problem orientation, the lack of clarity in terms of their executive responsibility meant that they ratified plans rather than contributed to the formulation of plans. In addition, social workers recognised case conferences as a forum in which they could obtain specialist opinions. The use of the case conference as an information gathering body and an opportunity to get the views of experts — for example psychiatrists, and educational psychologists — often led to the apparent paradox by which social workers and their team leaders would appear to play only a minor role at the meetings themselves, even although they could have instigated and orchestrated the occasion and would be responsible for carrying forward the recommendations and decisions of the meeting.

The sampled children's cases were rarely the subject of discussion at supervision sessions: in practice the allocation of time for social workers to meet with their seniors for supervision did not appear as a high priority. Where cases were discussed, discussion centred on bringing the senior up to date with recent active cases and obtaining endorsement of past action. Supervision rarely involved consideration of choices between possible alternatives for future action and the general content of supervision sessions seemed determined more by the readiness of social workers to bring forward and report certain features of their cases rather than the direction and guidance of the supervising senior.

In contrast, the impact of less formal means of discussing cases would seem to be highly significant and more pervasive in structuring social workers' decision making and planning practice. The support which social workers clearly derived from these as opposed to the more formal mechanisms may have implications for any attempt to change the nature of planning for children in care.

CHAPTER EIGHT
Remaining in Care, Decision-making and Planning

Remaining in care, unlike admission to and discharge from care, does not involve a change of status for the child and, as such, it is not an identifiable event in the same sense. In consequence, establishing when it was decided that a child would remain in care, far less who took that decision or on what basis, is not necessarily straightforward. Moreover, as will become apparent, remaining in care is not always the outcome of a decision, but may be the outcome of not taking a decision.

Table 8:1 below sets out the number of children who remained at the end of the study period, according to type of admission and length of time in care at the end of the study period.

Table 8.1
Children remaining in care at the study end: type of admission and length of time in care at study end

Length of time in care	Rescue from the family		Child behaviour		Service to the family		Other		Total	
	n	%	n	%	n	%	n	%	n	%
Less than 6 months	–		2*		–		–		2	
6 months – 1 year	17		25		3		3		48	
1 – 3 years	13		10		8		–		31	
3 – 5 years	13		4		–		1		18	
5 – 10 years	8		1		6		1		16	
Over 10 years	3		–		4		1		8	
Total	**54**	**44**	**42**	**34**	**21**	**17**	**6**	**5**	**123**	**100**

---

*These two children had left care during the study period but were subsequently readmitted and had been in care less than six months at the end of the study period.

However, each of the admission groups contained cases where the child's departure from care was fairly imminent. Overall there were 31 such cases, and although the numbers are small it may be significant to mention that in each admission group those likely to leave care represented approximately 25 per cent of the total group remaining in care at the study end.

In seven cases the adoption process was well advanced, five of these being cases which were originally rescue from the family admissions and in a further six cases, discharge was inevitable because of the child's impending 18th birthday, these cases being distributed evenly across the three main admission groups.

Apart from a further two child behaviour admissions where plans were underway to discharge the care order and transfer the young people concerned to the care of the probation service, the remaining cases represented children placed home on trial on care orders, and where, for a variety of reasons, there were plans to approach the court to seek revocation of the care order. These 16 cases were equally distributed between the child behaviour and rescue from the family admission groups.

This chapter is based on the 92 cases in care at the study end where there was no such likelihood of the child's imminent departure from the care system, that is the children whom social workers believed would remain in care 'for the foreseeable future'. Table 8:2 sets out these cases according to admission type and length of time in care.

As was the case with the overall population of children in care at the study end, rescue from the family admissions predominated with 17 of the 40 (over 40 per cent) already having spent over three or more years in care. The next largest group, child behaviour admissions, reflected a rather different pattern: 90 per cent of these had spent less than three years in care, and in fact almost two thirds had been in care for less than a year. On the other hand, precisely half (8) of the group entering care as service to the family admissions had been in care for three or more years. In the remainder of this chapter, each of the admission groups is considered in turn to explore the planning and decision-making process in relation to remaining in care.

Rescue from the family admission (n = 40)

The reader will recall that a characteristic of this type of admission was doubt about the prospects of the child ever returning home. On this basis, one might assume that, since approximately 30 of the 40 cases had

Table 8.2
Children remaining in care at the study end and likely to remain: type of admission and length of time in care at study end

Length of time in care	Rescue from the family		Child behaviour		Service to the family		Other		Total	
	n	%	n	%	n	%	n	%	n	%
Less than 6 months	–		2*		–		–		2	
6 months – 1 year	13		19		1		–		34	
1 – 3 years	10		8		7		–		25	
3 – 5 years	9		2		–		1		2	
5 – 10 years	7		1		6		1		16	
Over 10 years	1		–		2		1		4	
Total	**40**	**44**	**32**	**35**	**16**	**17**	**4**	**4**	**92**	**100**

*These children had left care during the study period but were subsequently readmitted.

been in care for more than a year, progress would have been made towards clarifying this point. In fact, in only 14 of the 40 cases did the social worker holding the case state that there was no question of the children returning to the care of the parents or parent from whom he or she had been removed.

In three such instances, it was possible to identify how and when this had become resolved: in two the child had become orphaned after entering care and had no home to return to, and in a third a teenage boy refused to return home or indeed have anything to do with his family. Otherwise, despite the fact that the children's social workers were adamant that the child would not return home, it was rarely possible for them to state, or us to identify, when this 'decision' had been reached.

In the remaining 26 cases, the social workers were less definite about what the future held for the child, stating that he or she would 'probably not' be returning home now or that they were 'not sure' what was likely to happen. It was clear from the case files that similar views to these had previously been expressed in most of the 14 cases where more definite statements were now being made. In other words, whilst it was expected, in varying degrees, that each of these 40 children would remain in care, there were few instances where this had been explicitly decided.

Analytically the decision that a child remain in care implies two earlier decisions: one that the child will not return home and the other that, for whatever reason, the child will not be adopted. In none of these 40 cases had there been conscious agreement on both these points. Adoption, far from being considered, was generally only referred to in the sense that passing references were occasionally made to the hope that the child's existing foster parents might ultimately wish to adopt. Rather, children remained in care because over time, it had come to be agreed or accepted that they would not return home.

The passage of time was perhaps the most significant factor in the process of determining whether such admissions would return home or not, as only with the passage of time were social workers prepared to make the transition from saying that a child *should* not return home to that he or she would not return home. For example, although choice of legal status on the child's admission to care was often said to reflect the feeling that the child should not return home, it invariably took several years of the child being in care before the social worker was prepared to state that this was what would happen, and then the fact that this feeling had existed since the time of admission was used in support of this outcome. The following two cases illustrate this point:

Cathy's case

Asked at the end of the research period whether seven-year-old Cathy, in care for almost four years, was likely to remain in care, the social worker replied: 'I think that's generally agreed. There seems little way she'll ever return home now. . . and I think that's probably always been the feeling. We did after all go for a care order, when it could have been voluntary'.

Philip's case

Speaking of four-year-old Philip, in care since he was eight months old, the social worker said: 'Time has proved the point here really. I believe there were reservations about the parents' long-term ability to care for him when he was admitted to care. Nothing had happened to make me change my mind about that and he's been in care more than three years now. No, he won't be going back home now'.

To decide that a child will never return home is a momentous step, not only for the child concerned, in terms of the implications for him or her but for the person or persons taking that decision, and it requires very careful consideration. As in other aspects of children's care careers, the data suggest that there was no departmental mechanism for taking this decision and, as such, the responsibility for resolving the situation rested with the social worker holding the case. To enable them to do this, social workers clearly felt the need for time to prove or to substantiate their case. The passive discouragement of parental contact following these rescue from the family admissions was one way in which social workers could demonstrate over time parents' low motivation to have a child back. The relative merits of this approach as opposed to taking an explicit decision and thereby restricting or denying parental access were highlighted by several social workers, one, for example, saying:

> You have to be very careful what you do. If you go as far as actually denying contact, then you are likely to have no case at all if the parents decide to test that.

It was also evident that in making the transition from 'should not' to 'will not' return home, social workers felt that they had to have an acceptable alternative to simply remaining in care, and it was clear that they did not view the prospect of remaining in care favourably. For example, it was said:

> It's very sad — there seems to be no alternative . . . she'll have to remain in care'.

> It's pathetic but it looks like he'll be in care till he's 18.

Adoption was not, however, viewed as a viable alternative. Despite the fact that there is a legal provision for dispensing with parental consent to adoption, most workers disposed of this option stating, 'The parents would never agree to that'.

On the other hand, long-term foster care did form an acceptable alternative. Thus, where the child was settled in foster care and the natural parents were no longer in regular contact with him or her, the future was viewed much more optimistically and social workers were also more likely to imply that it had been formally decided that the child would not be returning home. In these circumstances, the following was a typical comment:

> He'll be staying where he is . . . with the foster parents. That's his home now.

When the same social worker was asked if this meant the child would definitely not be returning home, the reply was:

That's right, the prospects for rehabilitation have never been good here and we've now decided this is where the future lies — with the foster parents.

Nonetheless as in this example, there was rarely any indication that a formal decision has been taken, only progressively positive reports of the child and the foster home and correspondingly negative reports of the parents' situation and involvement with the child. In other words, the expectation of a future with a new substitute family enabled the social worker to make the transition from strong reservation to return home to firm conclusion that this would not occur.

If parents did retain some degree of contact or the prospect of a substitute family was less certain, this transition was less likely to be made. In such instances, the question of return home was rarely entirely resolved and social workers, in time, resorted to encouraging parental contact which they had previously believed would be better reduced. With little security within care and often fairly tenuous links with home, the implications of the consequent confusion for children were often major. Social workers described several such children as displaying disturbed behaviour, which they attributed to the child's care experience. Brendan was one such case:

Brendan's case

When Brendan had been with his foster parents for about ten months, they expressed an interest in keeping him long-term. At the time the social worker recorded in the file: As the home situation is no better than when Brendan was removed, and the foster parents have said that they would like to keep him, we have agreed that he will remain there on a long-term basis.'

Shortly before the study start, the foster parents then asked for Brendan's immediate removal. By this time, Brendan's mother had remarried and since she had began to see Brendan again she asked if he could return home. This was eventually agreed on a home-on-trial basis.

A few months later, at the start of the research, the social worker said: 'It's too early to say yet but things do appear to be quite settled. Hopefully in time we may be able to consider revoking the care order. It's quite remarkable really. I never imagined he'd go back home.'

Comments such as these continued to be made over the next few months. Then, bruising was noted on Brendan, which both parents (mother and step-father) denied having inflicted. After Brendan had spent an overnight stay in hospital for medical examination, the social worker agreed, in consultation with her team leader, that Brendan could return home but that stricter supervision of the home situation would then be carried out.

Within a matter of weeks further bruising was noted. On this occasion, Brendan was removed from home and placed in a children's home.

In the final research interview, less than a month later, the social worker said: 'I can't see him going back — he's at risk if he goes back. But what's the future? He's already had a fostering breakdown. I feel all I can do is encourage the family to visit and keep up contact. But mother is already saying there's no point in that unless he is going back home. He is now a very disturbed little boy.'

In other words, although a marked feature of rescue from the family admissions was doubt about the child's prospects of ever returning home, such children do remain in care for considerable periods of time in the absence of firm decisions about their future. In some instances, this results in what may be considered a favourable, though unplanned, outcome for the child, long-term foster care, whilst in others it may result in long-term uncertainty and change. Whatever the outcome in individual cases, the fact that such children remain in the care system, and are expected to do so for the rest of their childhood, seems likely to be related to the absence of positive planning on their behalf.

Child behaviour admissions (n = 32)

In contrast to rescue from the family admissions, a feature of child behaviour admissions at the time of entry to care was the assumption that the children concerned would return home in due course, and, in general, this continued to be the expectation in relation to the 32 child behaviour admissions who remained in care at the end of the study. The fact that adoption was not considered for these children was, then, likely to be attributed at least in part to this.

Twenty one of these child behaviour admissions had formed part of the *into care* sub-sample and, as such, had been in care for at most a year. In five of these, social workers expected the young person concerned to remain in care until their 18th birthday: in two because medium to long-term psychiatric treatment was necessary and in three because the young people concerned had made it clear that they would not return to the parental home. However, the remaining more recent child behaviour admissions involved children who had retained contact with home, indeed a few were placed at home on a trial basis. Although the social workers dealing with these children rarely had explicit plans for them, they tended to be quite definite that the children would remain in care until school-leaving age at least. When asked in research interviews why they viewed the age of 16 as such a significant landmark, it was clear that social workers felt themselves to be influenced in this respect by what they thought the courts expected. As one social worker put it:

> I suppose it's learned behaviour really. Somewhere along the line courts must have consistently failed to revoke care orders on this type of case before they were 16. It's something we just assume they won't do — unless you've got a real little angel on your hands.

In other words, the care careers of child behaviour admissions were broadly defined at the outset in terms of length of time in care. This was reflected in the case conferences and other types of meetings held on individual child behaviour cases, the content of these meetings being placement-focused as opposed to being geared to consideration of the child's overall career in care. The older age of these 21 children at the time of their admission to care and, by virtue of that, the fact that they were unlikely to endure lengthy separation from their families by being in care also appeared to deter social workers from giving a high priority to whether or not and when such children would return home once they were in care. As the social workers on several of these cases put it:

> It's not as if they don't get home, they're often home on trial anyway.

The care careers of these 21 child behaviour admissions, in care for approximately a year, therefore suggest that child behaviour admissions in general remain in care on the basis of the assumption that such admissions do not leave care until at least the age of 16 years. It was only when this general rule was broken that decisions about children's care careers were more explicitly taken.

The remaining 11 cases, all from the *in-care* sample, represented a more varied group of cases. In some respects seven of them provided the opportunity for looking at what could happen to the 21 admissions just described after at least a further year in care. In three cases, the young people had been in care for almost three years and it continued to be said that they would remain in care till school leaving age at least, two of them, in fact, never having left home but remained at home on a trial basis. In a further four cases, school leaving age had always previously been mentioned but now it was said, 'We might as well leave it till he's 18'. In three of these four, the social workers had been genuinely surprised when the young persons made it known that they had no intention of leaving care to return to live with their parents, and the social worker had subsequently assisted them in moving to semi-independent situations. In the fourth case, the boy had returned home on trial but was unhappy about this move, was unemployed and had few prospects of finding a job. According to the social worker concerned:

> He's not in trouble or anything like that and you could argue that I should discharge the order. On the other hand, I don't see he's got a lot going for him and I feel he's not losing anything by being on a care order. . . he could even benefit. Being in care, I can provide money and that sort of thing, if he needs it'.

In these cases, then, whilst the young person's remaining in care was not necessarily the outcome of an explicit decision, it did entail responsive planning in the child's interests.

The remaining four cases of children from the in-care sample represent far less fortunate sets of circumstances. Although their entry to care on this occasion had been as a child behaviour type of admission, at ages ranging between seven and 12 years, each had extensive previous care histories as service to the family admissions, and in one case, as a rescue from the family admission also. Parental contact had diminished since they entered care to the extent that it was non-existent by the study start, and in each instance the family now said that they no longer wished to be involved with the child. All four were now in residential care although each had had previous foster care experience. On the whole, research interviews on these cases were characterised by recriminations about what had gone wrong in the past and lack of certainty about what could be done in the future. The risks implicit in the various alternatives, should they be available, were all-too-well recognised by the social workers concerned and other than in one case where a final 'effort' was being made to seek a long-term foster home with a view to adoption, each worker felt immobilised in attempting to improve the child's overall prospects. Needless to say, there was no plan or decision taken that these children would remain in care, but tacit acceptance that this was probably inevitable. As one of the social workers said:

137

What's the point of talking about it really. It doesn't get you anywhere. Everyone deplores what has happened but they can't or won't do anything about it. Try transferring this case or discussing the future — all you get is a stony wall of silence. Nobody wants to know — he's a casualty of the system and we can't take that.

Service to the family admissions (n = 16)

Whilst circumstances similar to those just described were not uncommon amongst the 16 service to the family admissions, who remained in care at the study end, it was here that there was most likelihood of identifying specific decisions about children's prospects of return home. It will be recalled that at the time such children entered care, there was little doubt that they would return home and their period in care was expected to be brief. At the end of the study period, however, there were a few cases where still it had not been decided that the child would remain in care.

With only one exception, the children involved came from the *in-care* sub-sample and as such only one had been in care for less than 18 months and most had been in care for over three years. All had been admitted to voluntary care in the first place although there were few now where a greater degree of legal security had not been obtained, in some by a resolution of parental rights and duties, and in others by obtaining a care order in matrimonial proceedings. The children tended to be fairly young, between five and 11 years, and in 11 of the 16 cases had entered care as part of a sibling group.

In general, the period prior to the decision that the children would not return home was preceded by diminishing parental contact, but the contact did not wither completely and was maintained by several visits over the course of any one year. However, many 'planned' contacts were not kept by the parents and a further feature of the run-up to considering the children's futures was reports from residential care staff of the children's disappointment and confusion at these unkept visits. Despite this, when the children's future was raised with the parents, they indicated that they intended to have the children back at some time in the future but were unable to specify when. In one case, the social worker reported that on each occasion over the last three years that she had raised with the mother when she would be having the children back, the mother replied 'in three years'.

138 The question of children's futures tended to be raised in the context

of the statutory review, in the written report of the social worker. How this was handled within the review, however, demonstrates again the widespread tendency noted in each of the study areas to remit planning for children to the social worker dealing with the case. Social workers tended to raise the issue by writing: 'We must assume that these children will not be returning home in which case we must make plans for their future;' or, but less frequently, 'We must consider if it is viable that these children will ever return home'.

In the former instance, social workers had already formed an opinion which was subsequently endorsed by those present at the review. In the latter social workers spoke of their concern and uncertainty about the magnitude of the decision to be made and their desire that it should be a *joint* decision. However, invariably, the question was not resolved at the review meeting but it was agreed that it did need further consideration. At subsequent reviews, this process tended to be repeated until such time as the social worker made a more explicit statement about what he or she felt should happen. In other words, whilst the decision was made 'official' by the review, it was taken at the initiative of the social worker.

Although the actual decision reached in such cases was based on a consideration of the likelihood or the desire of the parents to be able to resume care of their children, it was not necessarily this which had prompted the debate. Belief that children should be brought up in a family setting (and not in residential care) appeared to be a significant source of motivation. As one social worker put it:

> It wasn't doing them any good being there (residential home). They obviously needed to be in a family, so we had to consider whether we would ever be able to return them to their parents. All in all that seemed unlikely so we are now looking for a substitute family.

In other words, in some admissions various stages had to be gone through in the process of establishing whether or not a child remained in care. This process began with the premise that children should not be in residential care and progressed through to the conclusion that the child would not be returning home and the need to plan their future in an alternative substitute family setting. In some cases, this might have resulted in the search for an adoptive home and the children leaving the care system, but in these study cases it did not. Once more it was apparent that adoption was not perceived as an alternative to be pursued, and that substitute care was generally understood to mean foster care. In consequence, children remained in care. In the course of the study period, two cases underwent this process, both involving two-child sibling groups. Each case is recounted in detail to illustrate these points.

The Adams' Case

At the start of the study, the two Adams boys were aged six and eight years and had been in care for almost two years. They had had no regular contact with either parent for more than a year. The question of their return home had been raised at a review prior to the study start, but no clear decision had been taken. The parents had recently divorced and at the hearing the social worker had recommended and been granted a care order on both boys. According to her, this was because 'We felt it wasn't clear that the lads would return home and it was better to take this opportunity of being able to plan their future rather than just let the whole thing drift on'.

At the first review in the research period the situation of both parents was discussed. Little was known of the boy's father other than that he was planning to remarry, and it was said of the mother, with whom the social worker was in touch on account of a younger child at home, 'The difficulty she is experiencing with the one child for whom she is caring is such that we must conclude that she'll be unable to resume care of these two boys in the foreseeable future and we must make alternative plans for them'. At that review, alternative plans were not discussed but it was clear that it was anticipated this would mean moving from residential care.

At the next review, the social worker informed everyone that she had made initial enquiries of the fostering officer in her area and that no suitable foster parents were 'on the books'. The fostering officer had suggested that it might be necessary to advertise for foster parents specifically for these boys and that the social worker ought to consider whether she would be prepared to place them separately. This sparked off a lively discussion which eventually concluded with the agreement that the social worker should ideally seek a joint placement, but that the idea of individual placements should not be discounted.

At the end of the study period and after a further review, an advertisement had been placed in a local newspaper and a placement prepared to take one boy was being pursued. At that stage adoption had not been raised in any of the discussions on the case. Therefore in the final research interview and after the social worker had stated that the boys would remain long-term in care but hopefully in foster placements, she was asked if she had ever considered adoption in the case. She replied: 'No I can't say I have. I'm not sure if that would be appropriate here would it?' Asked why she thought this, she said: 'I don't know really I just never thought about it before. Nobody else has ever mentioned it and in any case, I can't see mother ever agreeing to that'.

Craig and Joanna's Case

Craig (9) and Joanna (7) were admitted to care at the request of their father. Their mother was unable to manage them and the family had accommodation difficulties. The children were placed together in a foster home. The parents did not visit them and, after they had been in care for almost a year, the parents approached the department for help in another matter, adding at the same time that they did not wish to have the children back. In consequence the local authority assumed parental rights and duties in respect of both children. A few months later, the foster parents requested that the two children be moved and they were then placed in a small residential home. They had been there approximately five months at the start of the study. The parents had been informed of the children's move and that they could visit weekly. They seldom did, and then did not pre-arrange the visit.

At the study start, the social worker said she thought it unlikely that either child would return home but stressed that no decision had been reached on this. Her own approach was 'to let it lie a bit really'. Several months later at a review, the head of the children's home expressed concern that both children were deteriorating in residential care and enquired why they were not in foster homes.

It was generally agreed that the children's situation was far from ideal and that plans for their future needed to be made. In consequence, it was agreed that for the next review the social worker would assess the prospects of return home and that the residential staff would draw up a profile of each of the children and their needs.

When approached by the social worker, the parents said that they would visit the children but they did this on only two occasions. When interviewed by the social worker about this, the father said little but the mother volunteered that she would like Joanna back but not Craig. The social worker attempted to impress on both parents that if either child were to return, contact would first have to be resumed. No visits took place.

At the next review the social worker relayed her discussions with the parents and added that she did not feel that Joanna should go home. Her opinion was generally shared as was her assessment that it was not necessary that both children be placed together. A discussion of the type of foster home appropriate to each child then followed, this eventually being interrupted by a newly appointed staff member present at the review in an observational capacity. He enquired whether adoption might not be appropriate. The reviewing officer, a senior staff member replied: 'No I don't think so. . . we are not in the game of splitting up families'. The point was pursued no further.

In the final research interview, the social worker reported foster parents had been found for each of the children and in both instances they were prepared to accept that the parents might visit. Asked if this meant that adoption had been discounted, the social worker replied: 'I haven't done anything about that. I can see there might be some sense in it but why go chasing after adoption when you've got foster parents. The point is we want to get these children into families'.

In several other study cases, this process had already occurred in the past but the search for foster parents had been unsuccessful, or the placements had subsequently broken down. In four of these 16 service to the family admissions this resulted in the separation of sibling groups of children and acknowledgement that the children would remain in long-term residential care. Because social workers were invariably unhappy about this, they tended to encourage any possible parental contact and in two cases it was clear that as the child reached his or her mid-teens, it was likely that he or she would follow the path of older siblings and return home.

The situation of children who were not placed in residential care was rather different and here again the influence of the child's foster parents was of paramount importance in determining the extent to which the decision that the child would remain in care was made explicit. Such children were commonly described as having been abandoned in care, that is, they either had no contact with their parents, or their parents, although in contact, showed no initiative to remove the child from care.

As one social worker put it, 'they parent by taking the children out for a few hours every other Saturday afternoon'. In these cases, the feeling that the child would not be returning home rarely transformed into a decision until such time as the child had been in care for a considerable period, or the foster parents volunteered that, if necessary, they were prepared to keep them. In the case records of these children, the following type of statement was noted, 'We must soon decide what is going to happen to this child . . .' and 'We must monitor how things develop and see if . . .' Then later, without further explanation, it would be said 'I think we now accept that these children are not going back home' and 'it's now generally agreed that this child won't be returning home'.

Summary

The fact that some children may remain in care for a significant part of their childhood does not necessarily imply that this has been a planned outcome on which firm decisions have been reached. By looking over time at the care careers of different types of admission, it is clear that such a decision is rarely taken or formally agreed. More commonly children remain in care because over time and for a variety of reasons, it becomes accepted that they will not be returning home. In this process the alternative exit from care, adoption, is seldom considered independently of whether or not the child's foster parents may ultimately wish to pursue this course of action. Children may thus remain in the care system by default.

CHAPTER NINE
Summary and Implications

This study originated from mounting concern that an increasing number of children were remaining longer in care, the question asked being, 'Why do some children leave the care system whilst others remain?'. In the design of the study, the diverse social, economic and political factors affecting families and in turn, whether or not children enter the care system, were recognised but regarded as only partial influences on the situation of children once they were in care. It was felt that at that point the agency factor was likely to become increasingly significant and for this reason, the study sought to examine children's care careers by focusing on the decision-making process in child care.

Each of the preceding chapters has concluded with a summary of its contents. In this chapter the main themes of the report are presented under the following headings: patterns of admission and care duration; the nature of social work engagement in child care and factors affecting care careers. However before this, two more general points are worth mentioning. First, it should be noted that whilst each of the areas involved in the study differed in certain important resource and organisational features, these did not appear to affect the overall pattern of decision-making observed to any marked extent. Indeed in this respect, similarities rather than differences prevailed across areas. Furthermore, although it is some time now since the original fieldwork was carried out, other studies on different aspects of the child care system have produced similar findings (see for example Millham *et al*, Packman *et al*, Fisher *et al*, all forthcoming) and current work suggests that such changes as have occurred highlight rather than negate the implications of this piece of work. The chapter concludes by considering these implications in relation to the further development of the child care service.

Patterns of admission and care duration

On the basis of looking at a number of children entering the care system and social workers' accounts of the reasons for this, the study identified three distinct admission types, a characteristic of each being the length of time social workers felt the children concerned were likely to spend in care. *Child behaviour* admissions, numerically the largest group of new entrants to care (40 per cent), tended to enter care as adolescents and were rarely expected to remain beyond the age of 16 years. The remaining 60 per cent tended to involve younger children, (those under eleven years): *rescue from the family* admissions accounted for approximately half of these, social workers viewing the prospects of these children returning home with some uncertainty; *service to the family* admissions entered care on account of what were viewed as temporary family crises and were considered to be relatively assured of returning home quickly.

On the basis of following the care careers of the children concerned for at least a year, we found that overall there did appear to be a relationship between duration in care and type of admission. It was also apparent that, whilst in general the rate of leaving care decreased the longer children had spent in care, between admission types this rate varied. For example, whereas 60 per cent of service to the family admissions left care within one month of admission and a further 25 per cent over the next five months, the corresponding rates for rescue from the family admissions were 20 and 17 per cent respectively.

The differential rates by which new entrants to care leave the system has implications for the composition of the in-care population at any one time. Although in applying the same admission-type categories to our sample of children already in care at the study start we were dependent on retrospectively collected data, this experience suggested that the in-care population, as opposed to the number of children entering the care system, is dominated by rescue from the family admissions. In the study sample, these represented 45 per cent of the total number, whilst service to the family admissions, who had been expected to return home rapidly, represented almost 30 per cent.

The data, therefore, indicate that certain types of admission may be more at risk of remaining in care than others. Although there may be issues concerning the appropriateness and quality of the care experience of child behaviour admissions, in so far as length of time in care is concerned, they appear to be less at risk, their age at the time of entry to care generally meaning that they leave care within three, and at most, within five years. The vast majority of service to the family admissions return home, too, often after relatively brief periods in care and certainly within six months of admission. However, counter to the assumption that all such children return home, the research has shown that those who remain more than six months are at risk of continuing within the care system indefinitely. On the other hand, as a group, rescue from the family admissions appear to be at great risk of remaining in care for lengthy periods once they are admitted. The fact that such children remain in care when doubt about the likelihood of their returning home has been a feature of their cases at the time of their admission implies, not only that this doubt was ultimately resolved by default, but that they were not provided with a secure or permanent alternative.

Social work engagement in child care

In terms of the opportunity to influence children's careers in care, the study confirmed that the key social services personnel were the social workers who held individual cases. Evidence of this was found at all stages of children's care careers. For example, despite the requirement that admission to care had to be approved by a senior member of staff, we observed, and indeed social workers were at pains to emphasise, the extent to which admission was, in practice, their decision. Not only did they state that their decisions were only 'rubber-stamped' by others but that they were able to structure information on a potential admission in such a way that admission became inevitable. In this respect, social workers acted as powerful gatekeepers determining who entered care. Whilst at subsequent stages in children's care careers social workers appeared less inclined to state that firm 'decisions' had been taken, as a group, it was they who assumed responsibility for overseeing children's situations and they, rather than any other social services personnel, who initiated changes. For example, examination of meetings and situations with a potential decision-making function highlighted that the view extended by the social worker tended to be accepted routinely, and that alternative views were rarely extended or explored. In this sense, individual case holders were in a powerful position to influence what happened to children.

Social workers' attitudes to care suggest that they would use this position to seek to ensure that children leave care as soon as possible. That social workers felt that local authority care was to be avoided and used only 'as a last resort' was indicated both by their reluctance to admit children to care and their resistance to confirming that a child would remain in care throughout childhood. The fact, too, that they admitted children to care with some notion of their prospects of returning home, suggested that subsequent social work activity would be directed towards achieving children's exit from care by the route most appropriate to their home circumstances.

The study found little evidence that this was so in practice. In the chapter on leaving care, it was shown that whilst the vast majority of sample children who did leave care did so by returning home, this rarely arose in consequence of rehabilitative work undertaken by the social worker involved. Indeed over the study as a whole, social workers seldom reported that they were taking specific actions or steps to work towards children returning home. More commonly they expressed only their 'hopes' that this is what would happen. They indicated that they 'kept in touch' with parents or were 'monitoring' the home situation but not necessarily working with them towards agreed common objectives, and ways of achieving them.

In general, the effects of their so-called 'neutral' stance were unrecognised and when, according to them, they were exercising no influence on a case, they were, in fact, creating obstacles to children returning home. The way in which social workers approached the question of parents' contact with their children reflects this particularly well. Even where it was expected or hoped that a child would return home, the significance of maintaining contact between children and their parents received little attention or priority.

On the other hand, the indirectly, and generally unconsciously, constructed barriers to contact created by social work action could be considerable when viewed from the parents' position. There was likewise little evidence of direct work being undertaken with children, and indeed several social workers voiced their anxiety if this appeared to be in prospect as they felt ill-equipped to do this. By not engaging in work with the family, when the family was already at least temporarily dispersed, social workers were in danger of facilitating the process of family fragmentation.

On the other hand, the chapter on remaining in care demonstrated that social workers held somewhat ambivalent attitudes to leaving care by adoption. This is not to say that adoption was not valued as an outcome for children in preference to their remaining in care but that as an outcome it was one considered not feasible in individual cases. Of some cases it was said that the parents would never consent to adoption therefore the possibility of adoption received little attention, whilst of others it was said that it was hoped that the foster parents might ultimately wish to adopt. Foster placements were, nonetheless, rarely made on this basis and social workers were themselves reluctant to raise the question of adoption with foster parents.

The chapter also highlighted that the process by which many foster placements attain long-term status is by short-term foster parents volunteering their willingness to keep specific children, already in their care, long-term. In this process, the option to pursue adoption is invariably by-passed, with the result that the existing care status is maintained, rather than new permanence achieved.

Factors affecting care careers

The paradox implicit in the above is perhaps the most significant finding of the research: whilst social workers are opposed to care and have scope to influence children's care careers, they rarely work towards children leaving care. In terms of the length of time children spend in care, this has the overall effect of increasing both the possibility that factors other than social work actions will determine what happens to a child and the likelihood that the social work influence on any one case is more by default than design.

In the chapter on planning, we have shown that although social workers use the vocabulary of planning, this is not to say that they engage in purposeful planning activity in relation to any of the three admission groups.

In relation to older children admitted to care by the courts on account of their behaviour, social workers held notions about the length of time children would have to spend in care before the court would be prepared to discharge the care order. In addition, stated plans tended to reflect current actualities rather that future possibilities, and were moulded in the first place by perceptions of what parents wanted or did, and subsequently by aspects of the child's in-care situation. In many respects, it was the wishes or needs of adults, not of the children concerned, which effectively determined whether or not children remained in care. For example in considering leaving care, it became evident that children generally returned home as a result of direct action by their parents, or less direct action by their foster parents in stating that they wished a placement to end.

148 The case histories of the few children adopted in the study period also

highlighted that the social work involvement in this occurrence took the form of responding to initiatives shown by foster parents, and to a lesser degree the child's birth parents. The significance of foster parents was further made apparent in the chapter on remaining in care: their willingness to keep a child or not, to adopt or not was repeatedly shown to affect whether children returned home, remained in care or were adopted.

The extent to which factors such as the behaviour and wishes of foster parents or parents can have a bearing on children's care careers appears in some degree to be attributable to the fact that in the absence of firm plans for children, social workers have no overall view to guide them in their dealings with cases and, in consequence, their behaviour typically takes the form of reacting to people and events. Of course in this process suitable outcomes may still result for some children. For others, however, it may mean remaining in care, arguably without sound reason.

Implications

The overriding implication of this report is that the risk of children remaining in care for lengthy periods is to a large extent created by the manner in which their care careers are managed within social services departments. Not only has this considerable resource implications in terms of maintaining large numbers of children over lengthy periods of childhood, but in human terms it is generally recognised that a local authority is unlikely to be able more than barely to fulfill the responsibilities of parenthood. Alarming numbers of study children described as disturbed or maladjusted had been admitted to care as very young children, some never having lived with their own families at all. Given, on the one hand, the depressing picture painted by this study, and on the other the existence in this country for some time of both a professional literature and a statutory framework promoting planning for children in care, what positive steps can the research suggest for the future? Three areas in particular are indicated.

First the research has undoubtedly confirmed the adage that the greatest risk is to take no risk at all. There is no reason, therefore, to suspect that a positive planning approach itself is in any way 'at fault'. Our findings do, however, suggest that some types of case are at one and the same time more in need of planning and at greater risk of not being subject to planning. The fact that our data on length of time in care point to a large in care population of rescue from the family cases is not to say that this is necessarily unchangeable. Indeed, given that social workers expressed doubt about the prospects of these children returning home at the point of their admission suggests that planning could be undertaken fairly immediately. By contrast, the need for attention on service to the family admissions may not be so immediate but some urgency is indicated if the child remains in care beyond six months. Establishing priorities along such lines may well facilitate the overall process of case management.

Regrettably the study did not directly address the question of why social workers behave in the manner in which they do. However in the course of the research a number of features were noted to act as barriers to planning. One such feature was the work situation of the social worker. Few would dispute the fact that child care work in general is fraught with difficulties. Not only are the questions which have to be addressed of momentous significance in the sense of the implications they may have on that most intimate aspect of people's personal lives, the family, but they involve situations which are often unpredictable and characterised by conflicts of interests. Taking decisions about such situations is therefore a risky business and to a large extent the appropriateness of a decision can only be judged with hindsight. This is the scenario in which social workers operate and it may well be that adopting a relatively reactive stance is social workers' way of coping with the uncertainty of these situations.

Chapters Six and Seven have indicated that a further feature of this scenario is the absence of any formal recognition of the risks which, in the event, social workers are expected to take. It was indeed apparent that in general social services departments remit responsibility for the futures of the children in their care to the social worker working with the case. In some instances members of the social work hierarchy deliberately avoided the attempts of social workers to have them share the risks. Needless to say the risk element cannot possibly be eliminated in child care work but this is not to say that it must inevitably have such a paralysing effect. The research raises the question of departmental responsibility for planning in child care and in this respect, it is likely that senior and middle managers may have to reassess their role in relation to child care work and the staff who daily interact with the clients of the service.

Thirdly whilst the notion of planning has generally been promoted within the social work profession, there has been little formal recognition of the skills required in this approach. Coping with the chaos of other people's lives and meanwhile responding to the interests of one child in particular requires enormous skills. Although the majority of social workers in this study were classed as generic social workers, it was clear that family and child care work comprised the vast majority of their caseloads and that they had considerable experience in this area. Nonetheless, the language they used and the behaviour they displayed suggested the need for skill development in child care. It seems evident that current professional and in-service training programmes are deficient in preparing the majority of social workers in the skills of counselling, support and negotiation, which are intrinsic to all child care work. It is to be hoped that both the profession and the employing authorities will give this matter urgent attention in the near future. All indications are that it would be wholeheartedly welcomed by social workers and in turn benefit their child clients and the families from whom they are separated.

One final point of a more general nature needs to be made before concluding. This study was concerned with children once they were admitted to care and did not deal with that other important aspect of child care work, prevention. However, by all accounts considerably more effort is focused on preventing children entering care than on facilitating their exit from it. This may indicate that the time has come to re-assess child care provision and service as a whole. Care need not be a bad thing — it is a service valued by many parents and children who use it in preference to other alternatives offered by social services departments. What is to be avoided is long-term drift in care and it is to this that the concept of prevention needs to be applied, not care *per se*.

APPENDIX
Supplementary tables referred to in the text.

Table A2.1
The 114 workers of the 185 children's cases: qualification, experience and job titles.

Years of experience	Qualified workers		Unqualified workers		Total	
	No.	%	No.	%	No.	%
Less than 1 year	4	5	6	19	10	9
1 – 2 years	9	11	4	13	13	11
2 – 3 years	11	13	5	16	16	14
3 – 4 years	15	18	1	3	16	14
4 – 5 years	10	12	2	6	12	11
5 – 10 years	16	19	6	20	22	19
More than 10 years	18	22	7	23	25	22
Total	**83**	**100**	**31**	**100**	**114**	**100**

Job Title						
Student	0	0	2	7	2	2
Social work assistant	0	0	6	19	6	5
Social worker	61	74	23	74	84	74
Senior case worker/senior social worker	11	13	0	0	11	10
Team leader/acting team leader	7	8	0	0	7	6
Fostering/adoption officer	4	5	0	0	4	3
Totals	**83**	**100**	**31**	**100**	**114**	**100**

Table A3:1

The 114 new admissions: admission type and age

	Child behaviour		Rescue from the family		Service to family		Other		Total	
	n	%	n	%	n	%	n	%	n	%
Under 5 years	–	–	17	50	12	43	3	43	32	28
5 – 11 years	–	–	12	35	12	43	1	14	25	22
Over 11 years	45	100	5	15	4	14	3	43	57	50
Total	45	100	34	100	28	100	7	100	114	100

Table A3:2

The 114 new admissions: admission type and sex

	Child behaviour		Rescue from the family		Service to family		Other		Total	
	n	%	n	%	n	%	n	%	n	%
Boys	30	67	20	59	15	54	5	71	70	61
Girls	15	33	14	41	13	46	2	29	44	39
Total	45	100	34	100	28	100	7	100	114	100

Table A3:3

The 114 new admissions: admission type and legal status at admission

	Child behaviour		Rescue from the family		Service to family		Other		Total	
	n	%	n	%	n	%	n	%	n	%
Voluntary care	16	35	19	56	28	100	7	100	70	61
Compulsory care	29	65	15	44	0	0	0	0	44	39
Total	45	100	34	100	28	100	7	100	114	100

In Care

Table A3:4
The 114 new admissions: admission type and anticipated length of time in care according to social worker

	Child behaviour		Rescue from the family		Service to the family		Other		Total	
	n	%	n	%	n	%	n	%	n	%
Few days maximum	2	4	1	3	–	–	–	–	3	3
Within 1 week	–	–	–	–	7	25	–	–	7	6
Within 2 weeks	–	–	–	–	5	18	–	–	5	4
Within 1 month	–	–	1	3	9	32	–	–	10	9
Within 6 months	–	–	1	3	2	7	–	–	3	3
Approximately 1 year	–	–	1	3	2	7	4	57	7	6
Probably till school leaving age	23	52	–	–	–	–	–	–	23	20
Till at least 16 years	14	31	3	9	–	–	1	14	18	16
Probably long-term care	–	–	11	32	1	4	–	–	12	10
Not sure	6	13	16	47	2	7	2	29	26	23
Total	**45**	**100**	**34**	**100**	**28**	**100**	**7**	**100**	**114**	**100**

Bibliography

Adcock M (1980a) 'Dilemmas in planning long-term care', in TRISELIOTIS J P (Ed) 1980 *New Developments in Foster Care and Adoption*, Routledge and Kegan Paul.

Adcock M (1980b) 'Social work dilemmas', in ADCOCK M and WHITE R (Eds) *Terminating Parental Contact*, Assocation of British Adoption and Fostering Agencies.

Aldgate J (1976) 'The child in care and his parents', *Adoption and Fostering* no 84 pp 29-40.

Bainbridge J (1973) *Children Who Wait in Islington*, A report for the Adoption and Fostering Working Party, Islington, Social Services Department.

Bayley M (1973) *Mental Handicap and Community Care*, Routledge and Kegan Paul.

Brown P (1974) *Ending the Waiting: 1, which child and what plan?*, Association of British Adoption and Fostering Agencies.

Bryce M E and **Ehlert R C** (1971) '144 foster children', *Child Welfare* vol 50 no 9 pp 499-503.

Cherniss C (1980) *Staff Burnout: Job Stress in The Human Services*, Sage.

Cooper C (1980) 'Paediatric aspects', in ADCOCK M and WHITE R (Eds) *Terminating Parental Contact*, Association of British Adoption and Fostering Agencies.

Curtis S (1981) 'Foster care drift', *New Society* vol 55 no 949. pp 144-145.

Davis L (1982) 'How long do we tolerate this nonsense?', *Community Care* no 393 p 15.

Davies B, Barton A and **McMillan I** (1972) *Variations in Children's Services among British Urban Authorities*, Bell.

Department of Health and Social Security (1976) *Guide to Fostering Practice*, HMSO.

Department of Health and Social Security (1981) *A Study of the Boarding Out of Children.*

Department of Health and Social Security (1982) *Child Abuse: A Study of Inquiry Reports 1973-1984*, HMSO.

Department of Health and Social Security (1984) *Review of Children in Care of Local Authorities*, A consultative document.

In Care

Drezner S N (1973) 'The emerging art of decision-making', *Social Casework* vol 54 no 1 pp 3-12.

Fanshel D (1971) 'The exit of children from foster care: an interim research report', *Child Welfare* vol 50 no 2 pp 65-81.

Fisher M, Marsh P and **Phillip D** *In and out of Care*, Batsford (forthcoming).

Goldberg E M, Mortimer A and **Williams B T** (1970) *Helping the Aged. A Field Experiment in Social Work*, Allen and Unwin.

Goldberg E M and **Warburton R W** (1979) *Ends and Means in Social Work*, Allen and Unwin.

Gottesfeld H (1970) *In Loco Parentis: A Study of Perceived Role Values in Foster Home Care*, New York, Jewish Child Welfare Association.

Hall A S (1974) *The Point of Entry*, Allen and Unwin.

Hilgendorf L (1981) *Social Workers and Solicitors in Child Care Cases*, HMSO.

Hoelgaard S (1984) *The Foster Care Triad: Structure and Process*, unpublished PhD Thesis, University of Cambridge.

Holman R (1970) 'Combating social deprivation' in HOLMAN R (ed) *Socially Deprived Families in Britain*, Bedford Square Press.

Holman R (1976) *Inequality in Child Care*, Child Poverty Action Group.

Home Office (1970) *Adoption of Children*, HMSO.

Home Office and **Scottish Education Department** (1972) *Report of the Departmental Committee on the Adoption of Children*, HMSO.

House of Commons Social Services Committee (1984) *Second Report . . . Session 1983-1984: Children in Care . . .*, HMSO. (Chairman: Renee Short).

Imber V (1977) *A Classification of the English Personal Social Services Authorities*, HMSO.

Jenkins S (1967) 'Duration of foster care: some relevant antecedent variables', *Child Welfare* vol 46 no 8 pp 450-455.

Lipsky M (1980) *Street-Level Bureaucracy*, New York: Russell Sage Foundation.

Maas H S and **Engler R E** (1959) *Children in Need of Parents*, New York, Columbia University Press.

McGrath M (1977) *Children in Care Survey*, Chester, Cheshire County Council Social Services Department.

Mapstone E L G (1969). 'Children in care', *Concern* no 3 pp 23-28.

Merton R K and **Kendall P L** (1955) 'The focussed interview' in LAZARSFELD P F and ROSENBERG M (ed). *The Language of Social Research*. New York, Collier Macmillan.

Millham S, Bullock R, Hosie K and **Haak M** *Children lost in Care: The Family Contacts of Children in Care*, Gower. (forthcoming)

Morris C (1984) *The Permanency Principle in Child Care Social Work*, Norwich University of East Anglia in association with *Social Work Today*.

Murphy H B M (1968) 'Predicting duration of foster care', *Child Welfare* vol 47 no 2 pp 76-84.

Neilson J (1976) *Older Children Need Love Too, Association of British Adoption and Fostering Agencies.*

Packman J (1968) *Child Care: Needs and Numbers,* Allen and Unwin.

Packman J, Randall J and **Jacques N** *Who Needs Care? Social Work Decisions about Children,* Oxford, Blackwell. (forthcoming)

Page R and **Clark G** (1977) *Who Cares? Young People in Care Speak Out,* National Children's Bureau.

Parker R (1971) *Planning for Deprived Children,* Harpenden, National Children's Home.

Pringle M L K (1980) *The Needs of Children,* 2nd ed Hutchinson.

Prosser H (1976) *Perspectives on Residential Child Care,* Windsor, NFER Pub Co.

Prosser H (1978) *Perspectives on Foster Care,* Windsor, NFER Pub Co.

Rowe J and **Lambert L** (1973) *Children Who Wait,* Association of British Adoption Agencies.

Satyamurti C (1981) *Occupational Survival,* Oxford, Blackwell.

Schaffer H R and **Schaffer E B** (1968) *Child Care and the Family: A Study of Short-Term Admission to Care,* Bell.

Simon H A (1957) *Administrative Behaviour,* New York, Macmillan.

Sinclair R (1982) *'Include them out?',* Community Care no 424 pp 18-19.

Smith D (1965) 'Front line organisation of the State Mental Hospital', *Administrative Science Quarterly* vol 10 pp 381-99.

Smith G (1970) *Social Work and the Sociology of Organisations,* Routledge and Kegan Paul.

Thoburn J (1980) *Captive Clients. Social Work with Families of Children Home on Trial,* Routledge and Kegan Paul.

Thorpe R (1974) 'Mum and Mrs So-and-So', *Social Work Today* vol 4 no 22 pp 691-5.

Turner W (1980) 'Waiting in foster care', *Adoption and Fostering* no 102 pp 17-21.

Webber R and **Craig J** (1976) Which local authorities are alike? *Population Trends* no 5 pp 13-19.

Wedge P and **Prosser H** (1973) *Born to Fail?* Arrow.